THE BURNED OUT PHYSICIAN

T0384498

Burnout is a major psychological and physical health-related problem for workers in all fields, but especially for those in the fast-paced and rapidly changing world of healthcare. Burnout has severe consequences for patients, including medical error, and is a leading contributing cause of depression and suicide among healthcare workers. Organizational science is just beginning to be applied in earnest to physician burnout and patient safety, and holds several potential keys to addressing these concerns. *The Burned Out Physician* is for two groups: healthcare workers (especially physicians) and patients (indeed, all of us). Physicians will use this book to get an accurate picture of what they are experiencing and how to change it, and patients will use this book to see what their healthcare providers are experiencing and learn how to help and/or protect themselves. The volume includes a checklist of burnout symptoms, and crucially a list of solutions as part of an active effort to solve the burnout crisis.

JOHN E. KELLO is a professor of industrial-organizational psychology at Davidson College, with a graduate faculty associate appointment to the doctoral program in organizational science at the University of North Carolina-Charlotte. Additionally, he is president of and senior consultant with J. E. Kello & Associates, Inc., an organization development consulting firm that serves a national list of clients. He has published more than a hundred articles in professional journals dealing with the creation of a "positive safety culture" and with the design and implementation of organizational training systems for high reliability organizations.

JOSEPH A. ALLEN is a professor of industrial and organizational psychology at the University of Utah. He directs the Center for Meeting Effectiveness at the Rocky Mountain Center for Occupational and Environmental Health. Dr. Allen has consulted for more than 500 nonprofit and for-profit organizations. He has published more than 150 papers in academic outlets, with his research focusing on three major areas of inquiry: the study of workplace meetings, organizational community engagement, and occupational safety and health.

THE BURNED OUT PHYSICIAN

Managing the Stress and Reducing the Errors

JOHN E. KELLO

Davidson College

JOSEPH A. ALLEN

University of Utah

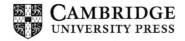

CAMBRIDGE
UNIVERSITY PRESS

CAMBRIDGE
UNIVERSITY PRESS

University Printing House, Cambridge CB2 8BS, United Kingdom

One Liberty Plaza, 20th Floor, New York, NY 10006, USA

477 Williamstown Road, Port Melbourne, VIC 3207, Australia

314–321, 3rd Floor, Plot 3, Splendor Forum, Jasola District Centre, New Delhi – 110025, India

103 Penang Road, #05-06/07, Visioncrest Commercial, Singapore 238467

Cambridge University Press is part of the University of Cambridge.

It furthers the University's mission by disseminating knowledge in the pursuit of education, learning, and research at the highest international levels of excellence.

www.cambridge.org
Information on this title: www.cambridge.org/9781316511466
DOI: 10.1017/9781009052795

First published 2022

A catalogue record for this publication is available from the British Library.

ISBN 978-1-316-51146-6 Hardback
ISBN 978-1-009-05591-8 Paperback

Cambridge University Press has no responsibility for the persistence or accuracy of URLs for external or third-party internet websites referred to in this publication and does not guarantee that any content on such websites is, or will remain, accurate or appropriate.

John: To my family and to the many teachers and students who have taught me
Joe: To Joy

Contents

Figures and Tables

Figures

Tables

Preface

Joe Allen: A few years ago, while receiving a relatively routine blood draw, I overheard the following conversation:

PHYSICIAN: I'm so tired.
NURSE: Tell me about it.
PHYSICIAN: I just need to survive the day.
NURSE: Sure, and then enter electronic records after the kids go to bed.
PHYSICIAN: Don't remind me. Can we really keep going like this?

And then they passed out of earshot. A patient overhearing that conversation might become somewhat nervous. Perhaps worried a bit about the physician or the nurse. Perhaps a little worried about the quality of care, the possibility of an error, and so on.

As an organizational scientist, I found this to be a fascinating interaction between colleagues at work. Until then, the possibility of healthcare workers – particularly physicians – being tired, burned out, or used up by their work never seriously crossed my mind. However, in hindsight, the classic telltale signs of burnout were more than present in that exchange: going into survival mode, feeling as if you cannot keep going. Those are expressed across so many industries. Now we had a new target to explore.

John Kello: A few years ago, I had cataract surgery. Over the half hour or so I spent being prepped for the surgery, several medical personnel checked in on me. Each one asked me my name, then checked the bracelet on my wrist for confirming identification, then asked me what procedure we were doing that day (ah ... cataract surgery), and then which eye we were doing today (um ... right eye). When I responded, each nurse, anesthesiologist, doctor, and whomever else (by that time the meds were kicking in, so who knows who else checked on me) put a Sharpie mark over my right brow. As a behavioral scientist and organizational consultant with a deep background in occupational safety, I understood the purpose of this ritual. These healthcare providers were doing everything in their power to avoid a wrong-patient, wrong-procedure, or wrong-site surgery. This and similar incidents in my contact with the healthcare enterprise, such as routine blood draws, minor hand surgery, colonoscopy, and other procedures, had shown the same double-check and triple-check processes in action.

In the last five years or so, I have broadened my research and consulting focus in occupational safety to include patient safety. This research and practice led inevitably to studies of the reasons for avoidable medical error, which in turn led inevitably to studies of burnout in physicians and other healthcare providers.

***

Joe and John have collaborated on numerous research and consulting projects in the broad area of organizational science. We have coauthored research articles and book chapters on several topics relating to organizational effectiveness. We recognized quite a while ago that we both shared an interest in safety in a variety of settings, including in healthcare. We decided that a thorough review of factors affecting safety in healthcare, especially patient safety, was a valuable effort we could and should undertake. So we delved into current data on patient safety, medical error, and burnout.

A preliminary search of the literature led both of us to some eye-catching and, to some extent, scary statistics concerning burnout among physicians. For example, in national surveys, around 44 percent of physicians say they personally experience burnout, and as many as 96 percent of medical professionals agree it's an issue for them. Further, 40 percent of physicians say they are reluctant to seek mental health treatment for burnout, and 41 percent of medical professionals choose to isolate themselves to deal with burnout on their own. Physician burnout costs up to $6.3 billion annually in the United States alone due to turnover and medical errors (Clark, 2020). While anyone can experience burnout under certain conditions, the extent of the problem among healthcare providers qualifies it as a true crisis that began long before the spring of 2020.

As we were beginning to research physician burnout and medical error, and preparing to begin writing this book, COVID-19 suddenly emerged and the coronavirus was soon declared a global pandemic, infecting millions and killing hundreds of thousands. This major catastrophe only made our research even more timely and important for our readers. Physicians and other medical providers on the front lines bore the brunt of the efforts to contain the pandemic, all while seeing sickness and death at levels untold in our lifetimes. That has continued. Patients who were scheduled for surgeries and other treatments were made to wait; in some of these cases, lives were lost due to delays in care as the pandemic raged on. In addition to the direct health impact of the pandemic, millions of workers around the globe were suddenly out of work, experiencing heightened job insecurity or job loss. For a host of reasons the pandemic has created a massive surge in mental health, domestic violence, and drug-related problems, all of which have added to the workload of healthcare providers during and likely after the crisis, whenever that "after" comes.

Many healthcare providers who were not on the front lines caring for COVID-19 patients experienced a sudden dramatic loss in business and revenue, to the point that many private practices shut down, and those that were still able to operate experienced furloughs and layoffs. Major hospital systems are still dealing with similar stresses from astonishing drops in their revenue. In short, the pandemic took a preexisting problem of physician burnout, challenging as that was, and dramatically increased it for all involved in healthcare.

Summing up, while burnout among physicians and other healthcare providers was already at a crisis level and growing before COVID-19, the pandemic has dramatically increased the risk for all involved at any level of the healthcare delivery enterprise. While our focus in this book is largely on the burnout crisis as it gradually evolved and became more visible over recent decades, the pandemic and its effects will be highlighted throughout the book, partly to illustrate the kinds of causal factors that create burnout, but also as a backdrop to a global healthcare system seriously in need of support/resources and, indeed, in need of major change, more so now than ever.

The purpose of this book is to first explore burnout in general before diving into the experience of burnout for physicians and other medical workers. We believe it is a must-read for every physician, both to help them understand what they are likely to experience, pre-, during, and post-pandemic, and to provide relevant informational resources based in medical and behavioral science research to help them manage their stress and reduce their risk of burnout. We believe it is a must-read too for other healthcare providers, including nurses and pharmacists, who, as our research revealed, are under the same stresses and the same risk of burnout as physicians. We also believe it is an important read for every patient, indeed for all of us. Patients need to know the pressure physicians and other medical care professionals are under so they can be their own advocate, and be more proactive, more knowledgeable, and more understanding when working with their care team. Finally, our hope is that healthcare system leaders at the top of their organizations and at the national level will read this book, particularly the chapters on potential solutions at the systems level, and go further to provide the resources that are sorely needed to stem the tide of burnout among their people, with its potentially devastating consequences to them and their patients. Those leaders are positioned to have the greatest impact on how healthcare is delivered and to make changes in policy that can benefit everyone involved in healthcare as a provider and/or as a recipient and, therefore, can benefit all of us.

REFERENCE

Clark, M. (2020, October 14). 30+ shocking physician burnout statistics you'll never believe. Retrieved March 2, 2021, from https://etactics.com/blog/physician-burnout-statistics.

Acknowledgments

A special thank you goes out to our medical care providers, both those who care for us and those we interviewed for this volume. We must also express our appreciation for the many medical researchers whose work we drew on to provide much of the evidence we present here. Without all of you, this book would not have come alive. We are extremely grateful for the efforts of our research manager, Emilee Eden, in assembling the final volume. Finally, we want to express our appreciation to the University of Utah and Davidson College for their support of our efforts; we are privileged to work there.

CHAPTER I

The Psychology of Burnout

It's an overwhelming sense of falling further behind, of "lagging behind the pace car."

—Professor at a major medical school

Overworked . . . fatigued . . . no energy . . . not enough sleep! We are supposed to be limited to sixteen hours a day in the hospital, but sometimes it's much longer.

—Medical student

Tired . . . exhausted . . . depressed . . . anxious . . . no energy . . . a sense that "something's not right" . . . always rushed at work, no time to double-check.

—Pharmacist

Symptoms of burnout are commonplace among many physicians and other healthcare professionals. This fact is both unfortunate and unsurprising; after all, healthcare providers are tasked with the care of patients who are physically, mentally, and/or emotionally compromised. These patients often understandably focus on the bedside manner of their physician or the level of personal care provided by a nurse, but what often goes unrecognized and unappreciated is the effort that a healthcare provider puts toward maintaining a generally positive and empathic persona regardless of their actual feelings. The fatigue associated with sustaining these caring personas is what motivated some of the earliest work on the concept of burnout.

At this point, you may be asking what exactly burnout *is*. "Burnout" is a commonly applied term used colloquially to express being tired or overworked, or worn out from too much of the same thing over and over. In popular culture and everyday conversations you may hear statements like those below:

- "We binge-watched *Game of Thrones* this weekend, and I am really burned out on it."
- "Not burgers again for dinner. I'm so burned out on burgers."

• "I'm so burned out on going to the movies. Let's just stay home and chill."

Burnout, however, is more than a simple feeling of tiredness. True burnout is a specific condition with a history of careful study. Let's move away from the layperson's use of the term to define it from a scientific perspective.

The World Health Organization defines burnout as "a syndrome conceptualized as resulting from chronic workplace stress that has not been successfully managed" (WHO, 2019). In other words, burnout occurs when the stress encountered at work exceeds the cognitive, physical, and emotional resources of an individual to maintain their effort, performance, and personal well-being while at work. The syndrome of burnout is multidimensional. Specifically, psychologists and clinicians who revised the *International Classification for Diseases* identified three defining dimensions of the syndrome (ICD-11, 2019), as follows.

1. *Feelings of energy depletion or exhaustion.* The exhaustion component represents the basic, fundamental, individual stress dimension of burnout. "I have absolutely no energy. Nothing left in the tank. I am drained. I am completely worn out." This aspect refers not only to feelings of being overextended but also to being depleted of one's emotional and physical resources.

2. *Depersonalization or increased mental distance from their job, including negativism and cynicism related to work.* The cynicism (or depersonalization) component represents the interpersonal-context dimension of burnout. It refers to a negative, callous, or excessively detached response to various aspects of the job, including the customers, clients, or patients one is there to serve. Typical statements indicating the depersonalization dimension are as follows: "I used to really care about my work. I was invested in it. At this point, though, I just don't care about my work or the people I have to deal with. I try to . . . but my enthusiasm is gone. I feel bad about it, but to be honest, I really don't care anymore. I'm all out of compassion. These people (clients, customers, patients) are just a number to me."

3. *Observed reduction in professional efficacy and/or decreased feelings of personal accomplishment.* The component of reduced efficacy or accomplishment represents the self-evaluation dimension of burnout (Alessandri et al., 2018; Shoji et al., 2016). It refers to feelings of incompetence and a lack of achievement and productivity at work. Those feelings may be accompanied by visible reductions in

effectiveness. This is what the reduced-efficacy facet sounds like: "I got into this career to make a positive difference, and I used to feel that I was making that difference. Now? I don't think I am really accomplishing anything at all. What's the point? Why bother?"

Whether you are a physician, a nurse, another healthcare provider, a patient, or a family member of any of those folks, this description of the three critical defining dimensions of burnout syndrome may sound familiar. These more specific definitions of the facets of burnout tell a story of what far too many professionals in many fields, including physicians and other healthcare providers, are experiencing daily.

Although this book focuses primarily on physicians and secondarily on other healthcare providers, this introductory chapter is intended to provide a more general background on the topic of burnout and will conclude with a self-diagnostic tool that anyone can use to see if they may be experiencing or are at risk of experiencing those debilitating symptoms of the burnout syndrome. If that tool signals that you either are experiencing burnout symptoms or are at risk of it, much of the balance of this book will likely be especially useful to you. If you are a physician, other healthcare provider, or a patient, the information we have gathered and summarized in this book very well may be a lifesaver. As we will emphasize throughout this book, healthcare providers are especially at risk for burnout, with potentially severe consequences to themselves and their patients.

Brief History of Burnout

Burnout was first identified and officially named as such in the research literature in 1975 by Herbert Freudenberger, a psychiatrist working in an alternative healthcare agency (Freudenberger, 1975). In 1981, Christina Maslach, a social psychologist who studied emotions in the workplace, published the Maslach Burnout Inventory (MBI), the first major measurement tool for assessing burnout (Maslach & Jackson, 1981). This inventory allows individuals to self-assess on the three critical defining dimensions identified in the *International Classification for Diseases* (sound familiar? Flip back a few pages for a review). Research on burnout as a phenomenon began in caregiving and service occupations (Maslach & Schaufeli, 1993; Maslach, Schaufeli, & Leiter, 2001; Schaufeli, Leiter, & Maslach, 2009). And decades before Freudenberger put a name to burnout, many professionals in human-contact-intensive, services-oriented professions lamented the emotional burdens of their work.

Burnout, of course, is not limited only to human services. Any job in any industry can lead to burnout, depending on heavy workload, long hours, low autonomy, and other factors. But there are certain consistencies in jobs that are especially associated with burnout. A recent survey ranked burnout-prone jobs in order of risk level: social work, emergency response, design, business development and sales, retail, medicine, and law (Montanez, 2021). A separate study placed medicine at the highest risk of burnout, followed by law and STEM (science, technology, engineering, and math; Stahl, 2020). We could cite dozens of such articles with different rankings, but each will inevitably list healthcare at or near the top of the list as a high-risk, burnout-prone profession.

What Are the Symptoms?

With our science-based working definition of burnout in hand, we will now explore some of the symptoms that those experiencing burnout can expect to see in themselves and/or in coworkers who are experiencing the syndrome or are verging on burnout. In other words, what does burnout feel and look like?

The symptomology and characteristics of burnout include a variety of cognitive, emotional, and physical elements. As one would expect, these symptoms map directly onto the dimensions identified by the World Health Organization and measured by the MBI (Maslach & Jackson, 1981; WHO, 2019). We summarize the main categories of symptoms here, and for those who wish to dig deeper into the symptomology of burnout (or any of the other areas covered in this and other chapters), we provide a list of references at the end of each chapter.

The most prominent symptoms of burnout include the following.

1. *Dysphoric symptoms center on emotional exhaustion.* Emotional exhaustion includes a general sense of unhappiness and a prevailing negative mood. Even things that would typically incite enthusiasm and a cheerful mood no longer do so. Emotionally exhausted individuals also commonly experience physical fatigue at a level that cannot be resolved by a good night's sleep (note that sleep disruption is a common, virtually universal correlate of the burnout syndrome; Ekstedt et al., 2006). Described as "a fatigue that is more than skin deep," the experience of emotional exhaustion includes biologically identifiable physical fatigue as well as mental fatigue that makes general alertness and complex thought processes challenging. The key term is exhaustion.

2. *Burnout symptoms include mental, behavioral, and physical deficiencies.* Many of the symptoms experienced by individuals with burnout are mental (cognitive), such as a lack of clear thought process, inability to focus and concentrate, being easily distracted, forgetting things, or missing steps in a procedure. Behavioral symptoms are also commonplace and may include choosing to distance oneself from people or expressing frustrations at minor hassles that normally are not particularly bothersome. Critically for healthcare providers, and central to the focus of this book, these behavioral symptoms can also include making errors. Physical symptoms in extreme cases are the familiar stress-related psychosomatic disorders, such as migraines, ulcers, or chronic hypertension (De Vente, Olff, Van Amsterdam, Kamphuis, & Emmelkamp, 2003; Peterson et al., 2008). Note too that current research has dramatically expanded the list of "stress-related diseases" beyond the classical list to include everything from the common cold to cancer. Excessive unmanaged stress predisposes one to a much wider range of physical disorders than those identified in the early research on stress.

3. *Additional observable behavioral symptoms of burnout relate to work performance.* Related to the previously described emotional and cognitive symptoms, another behavioral manifestation is disengagement in work activities, which in turn leads to inefficiencies and performance loss (Schaufeli, Leiter, et al., 2009). Tasks that are typically done without issue or error now become challenging and burdensome. Others within the workplace may begin to notice these changes. If severe, these deficiencies can result in major, even catastrophic mistakes, which in turn can trigger organizational and institutional sanction and intervention.

It is important to emphasize that these defining symptoms of the burnout syndrome do not occur in isolation, but come together and reinforce each other. For example, emotional fatigue and sleep disruption inhibit mental performance and mean that errors are more likely. More errors in turn add to the stress and emotional exhaustion. Withdrawal behaviors add to all the other symptoms. No matter how the cycle begins, once the symptoms become chronic, exhaustion, depersonalization, and reduced efficacy – the defining markers of burnout – will follow.

We want to emphasize that anyone, regardless of personality type, resilience, or any other psychological characteristic, can experience burnout. Recall that burnout is identified as a *work-related* syndrome, a serious condition to be sure, but not one that is classified as a form of psychopathology. Previous psychopathology or current psychopathology is not at all a necessary condition for these symptoms to emerge. Burnout is an "equal opportunity" problem that can affect anyone under the "right" working conditions. However, while we are all susceptible to burnout under the right conditions, previous psychopathology can exacerbate the symptoms and lead more readily to chronic burnout. Individuals who show the symptoms of burnout are disproportionately more likely to experience clinical depression, which is identified in all of the standard reference sources as a form of psychological disorder. Burnout is not in itself a type of psychological disorder, but it correlates with the condition of depression, and it is not always clear which leads to which. We will discuss more of this important topic later.

Given the symptoms of burnout and the reality that it impacts otherwise normally functioning people, you might ask a simple question: How do I know if I am at risk for burnout? To begin to answer this question, consider yourself as having a finite amount of energy and other critical resources. When your energy and other essential resources drop into the negative range, you might find yourself going into what may fairly be called "survival mode" at work. At that moment, you would be approaching burnout. You may be doing just enough to get by, waiting for the workday or workweek to end, hoping to be able to rest, recover, and return to work ready to go. But remember, one of the critical early warning signs and continuing challenges of burnout is sleep disruption. If you are beginning to approach burnout, available rest and recovery time might result in insomnia more than sleep.

Burnout, importantly, is not a sudden-onset condition like post-traumatic stress disorder brought on by a catastrophic event, or like sudden panic attacks. And the workload and lack-of-control issues that underlie and trigger burnout generally do not appear suddenly. Recall that the World Health Organization officially defines burnout as resulting from *chronic* workplace stress that has not been successfully managed (WHO, 2019). If an individual experiences a sudden emergency at work, marshals the resources to deal with it in the short term, and gets back to business as usual, that sudden extra demand on energy and other personal resources will not in itself lead to burnout. It may well lead to a temporary surge in the "stress reaction" otherwise known as the venerable fight or flight syndrome. There may be intense activation of the sympathetic branch of the autonomic nervous system, with a pounding heart, dry throat, tense muscles, butterflies in the stomach, and all the internal hormonal changes that underlie the felt stress reaction. It's true that in the aftermath of an especially intense sudden challenge, one might experience some level of post-traumatic stress disorder, with recurrent reliving of the event and anxiety-provoking flashbacks. But so long as those emergency events are uncommon, not extremely intense, handled well at the time, and not ongoing, a sudden spike in workload will not result in burnout.

For most people, the pressures that lead to burnout build gradually, as do the experienced symptoms of burnout. Individuals may be unaware that a gradual increase in their workload and the gradual decrease in their ability to control their workload are causing them to gradually begin to experience the early symptoms of burnout. In a sense, their "stress switch" is always half-on, but at a gradually increasing level of which they are unaware.

Remember the old adage: Question: How do you boil a frog? Answer: slowly.

Often it's easier to spot signs of burnout in others than in ourselves. When a colleague says, "We can't keep going like this," they may already be burned out, or at least clearly headed in that direction. Think about the symptoms of burnout that we outlined above. Subtle changes in overt, visible behavior can point toward inevitable burnout. Colleagues who distance themselves from others in the office, who become angrier or more argumentative, who fall behind on routine tasks, or who make atypical errors are showing warning signs of burnout. The key to addressing burnout in oneself and others is to be fully mindful of the symptoms and even the subtle changes that might indicate early burnout. A supportive conversation can help someone identify burnout before they suffer more serious consequences or leave the profession.

In this book, we will discuss ways to identify the signs of early or already-serious burnout, reasons why healthcare professionals are especially at risk, the effects of physician burnout on patient safety, and, finally, ways to put in place strategic interventions to mitigate and ideally even eliminate physician and healthcare provider burnout. But first, let's look at some of the primary outcomes of burnout, the effects of which are well documented in the research literature.

What Are the Cognitive, Job-Behavioral, and Physical/Health Outcomes?

A number of cognitive, job-behavioral, and physical/health ultimate outcomes are common among those who experience the symptoms of burnout. Again, and most fundamentally, burnout is a work-stress-related syndrome that should not be ignored in hopes that it resolves itself. It should be treated like any other serious condition in terms of urgency and availability of treatment options.

Cognitive Outcomes

Behavioral scientists have found that when a person starts to experience the symptoms of burnout, several specific cognitive outcomes arise in the form of impairments to the normal thought process (Bianchi & Schonfeld, 2016; Linden, Keijsers, Eling, & Schaijk, 2005; Peterson et al., 2008; Sandström, Rhodin, Lundberg, Olsson, & Nyberg, 2005). The following cognitive outcomes are broken out into three related facets. These impairments in the thought process are visible in the early stages of burnout as minor "misses," but they evolve into major problems as burnout builds over time.

1. *Impaired cognitive performance.* Chronic burnout leads to several types of cognitive performance impairment, including reductions in non-verbal memory, poor problem solving and decision making, and inconsistent prioritizing (Peterson et al., 2008; Sandström et al., 2005). In jobs where these forms of cognitive capabilities are required, such as every facet of healthcare, burnout results in immediate, often severe performance deficits. Think of this impairment in general as "not thinking clearly . . . forgetting something . . . missing a step."

2. *Cognitive attentional difficulties.* Cognitive attentional difficulties are challenges to the ability to be aware of stimuli in one's environment at a normal operating level. Individuals at varying levels of burnout lose their ability to fully maintain voluntary control over attention (Linden et al., 2005). Those with chronic burnout may be easily distracted, increasing the probability of errors during tasks requiring consistent attention, as most tasks in healthcare do. Think of the attentional facet as "I got distracted by X, now where was I with Y? "

3. *Depressive cognitive style.* Individuals experiencing burnout are also prone to develop what is identified in the research literature as a depressive cognitive style (Bianchi & Schonfeld, 2016). They develop dysfunctional attitudes, ruminate on recent failures or challenges, engage in self-blame, and make more pessimistic attributions about their environment than others. These trends may well help to explain, or at least offer clues, as to why burned-out individuals are so susceptible to depression. The positive correlation between burnout and depression is an issue critical to the health of the healthcare professional and the safety of the patients they serve.

Taken together, the various cognitive effects can be summed up as difficulties with focusing attention as needed, with effective problem-solving and decision-making, and with the ability to properly prioritize tasks. More generally, this dysfunction results in a greater likelihood of mental mistakes, which can translate to performance mistakes. Awareness of these deficits results in increased anxiety and (especially) depression, which adds to the stress that the individual is feeling.

It comes as no surprise that those suffering burnout show more pronounced cognitive performance decrements compared to non-burned-out individuals (Sandström et al., 2005). As with any of the outcomes of burnout, there are gradations to the negative cognitive effects. As soon as an individual feels any of the symptoms of burnout, cognitive deficits are at risk of occurring, and there is limited time before those deficits become apparent in their performance on the job and most likely affect cognitive ability and behavior outside the workplace as well. Remember that while the sources of burnout are work-related, the effects are not at all limited to the workplace. We are focusing here mainly on work-related outcomes, but as we will see, symptoms and outcomes can manifest themselves in any setting, including with the families of burned-out individuals.

Job-Related Outcomes

The diminished cognitive capacities will most definitely at some point result in job-performance declines. However, we will first address several additional job-related outcomes that occur as a result of burnout, as discussed by the pioneering burnout researcher Christina Maslach and the many colleagues and researchers who have been inspired by her seminal work through the years.

We review some of the additional major job-related outcomes as well as the overall performance decrement here.

1. *Reduction in positive job attitudes.* Burned-out individuals are less satisfied with and less committed to their jobs and organizations. Prior to experiencing burnout, individuals who are happy and committed to their work are more likely to have positive job attitudes that express themselves in a wide variety of constructive behaviors. They are more prone to engage in helping behaviors (e.g., offering to take on an extra task or staying late to help a coworker) and otherwise demonstrate increased engagement in work. Helping behaviors above and beyond the mere requirements of the job are termed

organizational citizenship behaviors or extra-role behaviors, and they are common in positive work cultures where people are not greatly at risk for burnout (Erks, Allen, Harland, & Prange, 2020). Similarly, high levels of employee engagement, where employees are deeply committed to their organization, their supervisor, and their teammates are common in positive work cultures where the risk of burnout is low. As a result of burnout, those positive job attitudes and the helping behaviors commonly associated with them are greatly reduced.

2. *Increase in negative job attitudes.* Not surprisingly, reduced positive job attitudes generally correspond to increased negative job attitudes. Physicians who become burned out will of course experience the defining symptom of cynicism and therefore be more likely to distance themselves from their work, particularly in terms of patient interaction. Additionally, thoughts of quitting a job become common and the negative job attitude becomes visible to others at work through a variety of verbal and overt behaviors, as evidenced by many of the quotes from the healthcare providers we interviewed for this book.

3. *Decrease in job performance.* A decrease in job performance is not just a reduction in productivity, but commonly includes an increase in errors on the job. In many occupations, a heightened number of errors might mainly pose a risk to profit through poor product or service quality. In other jobs, errors can result in injuries. However, in a field like surgery, an increase in errors from burned-out surgeons or others on the surgical team can have life or death consequences for patients. While perhaps not as starkly visible, errors from other healthcare providers can also have very severe consequences. We will continue to discuss the central theme of medical error and its relationship with burnout throughout the course of the book.

Physical and Health Outcomes

The many symptoms and outcomes of the syndrome of burnout interact and reinforce each other. In particular, the physical and health outcomes associated with burnout rarely, if ever, exist in isolation from cognitive and job-related outcomes. A person who experiences cognitive deficits, for example, is more likely to see the result of those deficits in poor performance on the job. A person whose burnout is accompanied by depressive symptoms (which is common) may experience physical symptoms that impact their health. We isolate these symptoms for purposes of analysis and discussion, but we must reiterate that they are all at play at any point in time.

The following physical and health outcomes have been observed in individuals as a result of ongoing burnout, regardless of industry or specific professional role. Research conducted in the early 2000s by Ekstedt and colleagues as well as De Vente and colleagues identified a number of negative physiological and health outcomes commonly associated with burnout, including the following (De Vente et al., 2003; Ekstedt et al., 2006).

1. *Increase in cholesterol and triglycerides.* Burnout appears to be especially closely related to risks to heart health. Burned-out men tend to show increases in their overall cholesterol, while women see increases in serum lipids. Prolonged, excessive, unmanaged job stress may have eventual long-term impacts on cardiovascular health for both men and women.

2. *Elevated resting heart rate.* Individuals experiencing burnout have a higher resting heart rate on average than those who are not overly stressed by their work. This may come as no surprise, as elevated heart rate is of course commonly associated with an increase in general stress. However, this is yet another concerning symptom for those in chronic burnout situations. It should be noted that according to existing data, blood pressure does not appear to be impacted by burnout, and research findings on elevated cortisol are mixed.

3. *Disturbed sleep or related sleep issues.* Disturbed sleep or other related sleep issues are among the most problematic issues related to burnout. Restful sleep is one of the main ways that we replenish our depleted physical and mental resources, therefore allowing us to cope more effectively with the stressors around us. We can see the challenges of sleep disruption in shift workers, whose circadian rhythms are continually disrupted by their work schedules. The challenges of shift work have been well documented for factory workers and first responders. But note that some healthcare workers such as nurses are shift workers as well. Burnout causes similar disruptions in the cycle of "normal sleep." The evidence suggests clearly that burned-out individuals experience more difficulty in falling asleep, more mid-sleep arousals, greater sleep fragmentation, more wake time, lower sleep efficiency, less slow-wave sleep (dominated by delta waves as detected in the EEG), and less REM (rapid eye movement) sleep compared to

those not burned out. Much recent research has been conducted on the distinctive REM sleep phase, finding that REM plays a role in memory consolidation and neurogenesis, or the process of formation of new neurons in the brain, especially in the hippocampus (Ackermann & Rasch, 2014). REM sleep is critical to the integrity of the overall sleep cycle. If individuals are explicitly REM-deprived (in sleep-research laboratories), they show substantial increases in REM at the next sleep opportunity (REM rebound). While less is known about the functions of slow-wave sleep (non-REM), sleep deprivation studies show that slow-wave sleep also rebounds.

> Any disruption in "normal" sleep is problematic. Without high-quality sleep, individuals can never fully recover from the stress of a previous day, much less the stress of the previous week or month. Low sleep quality helps drive the cycle of burnout, making it particularly difficult for the sufferer to ever fully recover. And, as we will see, one of the traditional, commonly advised stress-management strategies is to "get more sleep." For the individual experiencing burnout, that is easier said than done.

Taken together, the common cognitive, job, behavioral, and physical/health outcomes of burnout create a perfect storm. This combination of outcomes raises the likelihood that burnout will become chronic, especially for those who work in occupations with high workloads and other burnout-predictive factors.

Prolonged Stress at Work as the Primary Culprit

Let's pause and reflect on those work-related factors that are predictive of burnout. The common denominator and main culprit in the burnout formula is stress. It is the essential condition, the common denominator in all cases of burnout. The World Health Organization definition makes that point briefly and directly, calling burnout "chronic workplace stress that has not been successfully managed" (WHO, 2019). But what generates that workplace stress?

Excessive workload, short timelines, long hours, and other work demands add stress and therefore automatically increase burnout risk (Schaufeli, Bakker, & Van Rhenen, 2009). That is the case even when the workload is self-imposed and is definitely the case when the workload is imposed by others, leaving the individual with relatively little control over it (perceived control over the stressors being a major factor reducing burnout risk).

Constant interaction with others, be they coworkers, clients, customers, or patients, also adds stress. This stressor is certainly not limited to healthcare or other human services professions, however. While the earliest research that identified the syndrome of burnout was conducted in especially challenging, high people-contact work settings (Maslach & Schaufeli, 1993; Maslach et al., 2001; Schaufeli, Leiter, et al., 2009), any people-intensive, public-facing work is stressful in and of itself. Healthcare professionals are familiar with the need to maintain a good "bedside manner" regardless of one's true feelings and know how easily that exacts an emotional toll. However, teachers, retail workers, restaurant workers, and others of the same ilk also constantly deal with people and their needs, and also must regulate their own feelings and at some level "put on a happy face" no matter what. There is a research literature on so-called surface acting, the requirement to fake positive emotion even when that is not what one is feeling (Allen, Pugh, Grandey, & Groth, 2010; Grandey, 2000). Both Joe and John have directly contributed to this literature as researchers. Such surface acting requires effort and emotional labor. It is in itself stressful. Our research has shown that in, say, a common setting as a staff meeting when "higher-ups" are present (one's boss or boss's boss), meeting participants are more prone to surface act (expressing agreement or positive emotions when that is not how they truly feel) and that they experience such surface acting as stressful (Shumski Thomas et al., 2018). In sum, people-intensive work of any kind, by its very nature, requires some level of surface acting, which in turn requires emotional labor and is thus stressful.

Another work-related stress factor that can arise regardless of workload or people-intensity is poor relationships with one's boss and/or coworkers. Extensive research indicates that the most important relationship one has at work is the relationship with the immediate supervisor. The standard surveys that assess employee engagement contain many questions that ask either directly or indirectly about the quality of one's relationship with the immediate supervisor. Good relationships breed engagement and a positive work attitude. Bad relationships are stressful in and of themselves and magnify the negative effects of other job-related stressors.

Fight or Flight

How can workplace stress potentially lead to the burnout syndrome? According to stress research, when a potentially stressful situation occurs, the affected individual quickly makes a "primary appraisal" of the situation. "Is it relevant to me? If so, is it a potential threat to my well-being?" If the answer to those questions is yes, the individual makes what is known as a "secondary appraisal." "Am I able to cope? Can I handle it?" If the answers to the primary appraisal are "No, it's not relevant to me" or "Yes, but it is not threatening to me," then little or no stress reaction occurs. If the answer to the secondary appraisal is "Yes, I can handle this challenge," there is little or no stress reaction. But if the primary appraisal identifies the situation as a threat and the secondary appraisal predicts a failure to cope, then the stress reaction is activated. The situation is a stressor. A profound internal physiological reaction is then triggered. This is known as the "general adaptation syndrome" or the "fight or flight syndrome" (Selye, 1950).

Our bodies are exquisitely adapted to handle stressful situations in the short term. In the presence of a stressor, that fight-or-flight reaction that we share with nonhuman animals automatically kicks in. The symptoms of arousal that we feel are the result of the activation of several primitive regions of the brain, prominently the hypothalamus. That tiny structure (about the size of the last digit of your little finger) is the highest region of the autonomic nervous system. In the presence of a stressor, the hypothalamus activates the adrenal glands to release hormones into the bloodstream. These hormones shift the body's internal resources away from functions that promote long-term survival, such as digestion and the immune system, and toward functions that promote short-term survival, such as narrowing and focusing of attention, increasing heart rate and respiration, and tensing of the muscles. This automatic activation of the sympathetic branch of the autonomic nervous system and concurrent reduction in activity of the parasympathetic branch is accompanied by the experience of strong emotion. The hypothalamus is intimately interconnected with subcortical structures known collectively as the limbic system, which are strongly associated with our feelings of anger, fear, and other emotions.

In the first stage of fight or flight (McCarty, 2016), the hypothalamus directly neurally activates the adrenal medulla to dump catecholamines into the bloodstream. At the same time, the hypothalamus indirectly activates the adrenal cortex to dump corticosteroid hormones into the bloodstream, activating the pituitary gland directly to release a trophic hormone identified as ACTH into the bloodstream, where it has a slower but equally profound effect on the adrenal cortex. In the first stage of the stress reaction, called the "stage of alarm," the body and mind are as prepared for quick action as they can be. You are ready to fight or flee. If the fight or flight eliminates the stressor, the general adaptation syndrome has done its work, the sympathetic activation subsides, and balance is restored between sympathetic and parasympathetic autonomic arousal. What an ally for dealing with short-term emergencies!

But what if this response is ineffective in eliminating the stressful situation? What if the workload is still excessive? What if you have little control over it? What if there are more and more people you have to deal with and surface act with every day? What if the bad relationships at work don't get better? Then the initial alarm stage gives way to a second stage of "resistance." During that second stage the internal activation is less intense and likely not as noticeable, but it is still present. That's when "the stress-switch is half-on" and the body and mind are trying as best they can to cope. If the stage of resistance is prolonged enough, the result can be the third and final stage of the general adaptation syndrome, the stage of "exhaustion."

At the point of exhaustion, something breaks down and the individual may experience profound physical and emotional exhaustion, feelings of cynicism, feelings of ineffectiveness – in sum, the full syndrome of burnout. During the stage of exhaustion, the individual is likely to feel depressed and to make mistakes. In some cases, the individual is likely to suffer a serious psychosomatic illness, that is, a bodily breakdown (somatic condition) mainly as a result of stress (the psychological part). Stress diseases that have been previously identified include heart attacks, strokes, chronic hypertension, migraines, and ulcers, but today that list has dramatically expanded to include everything from the common cold to cancer. Stress is the primary culprit in burnout, and stress can indeed kill.

Whatever the contributing causes of the prolonged unmanaged workplace stress that underlie the syndrome, burnout is often self-perpetuating and is therefore difficult to reduce once symptoms have first appeared and have become intense. Let us turn to those who are at greatest risk for developing burnout and, from a general description of them, begin to paint a portrait of the burned-out physician.

Who Is at Risk?

There are two major broad categories of risk factors: environmental/ occupational and individual. The environmental and occupational risk factors are related to the nature of a job; different aspects of the work (e.g., resources and support) put people at risk for developing burnout. Individual risk factors are those differences between individuals that make some more at risk than others. These include personality as well as general demographics such as age, gender, and ethnicity. It is extremely important to note the following: while both are important, *environmental and occupational risk factors are much more strongly connected to burnout than individual-difference risk factors.*

To be sure, some individuals are more stress-prone than others and more likely to develop burnout than others, regardless of the situation. But critically, some environmental/work situations are such powerful triggers to burnout that they predispose almost anyone, regardless of their individual personality or other characteristics, to experience burnout. We will argue in the course of this book that given a choice between interventions or solutions that target enhancing individual capabilities (e.g., resilience/hardiness) versus environmental/occupational characteristics (e.g., caseload, pace of work, administrative burden), one must *always* choose the latter. If such a stark choice is not required, as is most often the case, one must *always* focus on both!

We provide here a list with definitions and examples of some of the more common risk factors across the two major domains of work-related and personal characteristics (e.g., Aydemir & Icelli, 2013). Research on burnout is ongoing and rapidly growing, so this is not intended to be an exhaustive list, but it does provide a starting point for understanding who is more at risk and who may be less at risk for burnout at work. And again, it lays the foundation for understanding why doctors and other healthcare providers are especially at risk (Amoafo, Hanbali, Patel, & Singh, 2015).

Environmental and Occupational Risk Factors

We outlined some of the general work-related sources of stress earlier in this chapter. Let's expand the list and explore them in a bit more depth and detail here.

1. *Low job control/autonomy*: the degree to which an individual has the latitude to decide what to work on, including both specific tasks and the timing of those tasks. Consider the contrasting examples of an assembly-line factory worker, whose work is routine and narrowly defined, and a college professor, who has complete control over significant parts of their work (e.g., research). The relative lack of autonomy in the job would predispose the factory worker to be more at risk than the professor.
2. *Workload*: the amount of work a person is asked or required to complete. All of the data point to workload as a central issue. It is problematic when the workload continually exceeds a person's ability to complete it. For example, when employees have to absorb the tasks

of colleagues who have been laid off in addition to their regular job responsibilities, their workload necessarily increases.

3. *Job demands*: these typically include workload per se, but also include the number and range of different types of tasks required of an employee, and the knowledge and skill required to perform them successfully (plus the training required in order to be able to do so). For example, the central job of the car salesperson is to sell automobiles, but a working knowledge of and understanding of human behavior and specific sales "closing techniques" are job demands for successful automobile sales people.

4. *Social support* (supervisor, coworker, friends, and family): the degree to which one's supervisor, coworkers, and leadership at work provide encouragement, helping behavior, empathy, and related expressions of social support for an employee. Social support also includes the degree to which family and friends outside work are encouraging and facilitative of work-related tasks and duties. A lack of social support – for example, lacking a confidant-like work colleague or family member with whom one can safely and openly discuss work-related problems – is strongly associated with risk of burnout. And as we will see, social support in general is one of the strongest general buffers against burnout.

5. *Job insecurity*: the degree to which employees feel their position in the organization is tenuous. Jobs that are seasonal or have a high turnover rate for reasons outside the control of the employee would be considered high in job insecurity and contributing to burnout. During times of major organizational change, especially when jobs may be at risk (such as during mergers or acquisitions, or during the COVID-19 pandemic, of which we will have much more to say), the general level of job insecurity is automatically higher.

6. *Pay structure*: how one is monetarily compensated for their work. In terms of burnout, compensation that is directly tied to billable work is associated with burnout (e.g., billable hours for lawyers or consultants or piece-rate pay for some factory workers). In such pay systems, time away from task costs the employee money. The temptation is to do more and more and more. The resulting heavy workload is self-imposed in order to increase compensation. As we will see, the prevailing fee-for-service or volume-based compensation system for many doctors automatically raises their burnout risk.

7. *Work-family imbalance*: the degree to which work demands and family demands do or do not receive equal and appropriate attention.

When there is an imbalance toward work, burnout is more likely to occur.

8. *Unrewarding career*: the degree to which a person feels their career or their job lacks meaningfulness for them. Some factory work, especially work done on the assembly line, may not be automatically meaningful and personally rewarding to employees. Punching out widgets for eight hours at a time is not automatically rewarding. In most cases, the concern about an unrewarding career is a lesser concern for physicians, but those in stereotypical "dead-end" jobs often experience this risk factor. As a sidebar comment, there have been active movements since the 1960s and 1970s to redesign assembly-line type jobs to be more "enriched," more team-based, engaging, and rewarding.

9. *Time pressure*: the degree to which the work has a high urgency factor due to either artificial or actual deadlines for critical outcomes. For example, servers waiting tables may have time pressure as their number of tables increases and/or customers express urgency for getting their food and drinks. Other industries have weekly, monthly, or annual cycles of times when the work is at a peak. Examples of such cycles include closing the financial books at the end of a month, quarter, or fiscal year; running flour mills at full blast during the holiday/baking season; running a paving business during the warmer spring and summer months; grading exams and term papers at the end of a semester.

10. *Role conflict*: the degree to which different aspects of one's job are at odds with each other. Requirements for one task may conflict with requirements for another task, rendering at least one of the tasks (maybe both) difficult or impossible. Imagine firefighters providing support to victims of a house fire while at the same time struggling to quickly extinguish the fire.

11. *Role ambiguity*: the lack of clarity around one's work tasks or objectives. Role ambiguity is surprisingly common in the workplace, regardless of the nature of the work. This phenomenon occurs when someone has not received a clear role definition and clear objectives, has not received necessary training, or has found that training was inadequate for the reality of the required work. Feelings of role ambiguity often coincide with feelings of burnout, particularly the facet of low personal accomplishment/efficacy. John and Joe have both had experience in facilitating team building sessions with work groups in a variety of industries, and in essentially every case, the

client groups had experienced a lack of clarity in "who does what and what is expected of me" in their teams.

12. *Job resources* (physical): the extent to which one is provided with the necessary tools for carrying out their work. For example, having enough respirators for all the ICU patients experiencing shortness of breath and low oxygen levels.

13. *Working with people*: We elaborated on this job factor in detail earlier. It is simply the extent to which the job/occupation requires one to interact directly with people. For example, office workers work closely with people both as colleagues (internal) and potentially as customers or vendors (external). People-intensive work has a unique set of work demands (e.g., professionalism standards) that are not necessarily defined in a job description (e.g., being polite, courteous, and kind to fellow employees and external stakeholders). As we discussed earlier, any people-intensive work automatically carries with it an elevated risk for burnout, especially as it requires surface acting, which in turn exacts emotional labor (see below).

14. *Emotional labor*: the degree to which the organization requires good customer service or empathy toward people who are demanding or may be suffering. Emotional labor may require individuals to express positive emotions and hide negative emotions, regardless of how they are actually feeling. For example, being a cashier at a retail store often requires smiling and providing friendly service regardless of whether the cashier may be having a bad day. The pressures can deepen depending on the occupation. Another example is a social worker who handles cases of child abuse or neglect and who may be required to express empathy and understanding repeatedly in an effortful, ongoing manner. Such an expenditure of effort and emotional labor may, in time, contribute in a major way to emotional exhaustion and burnout.

Individual Risk Factors

1. *Emotional stability*: refers to the degree to which one does or does not experience large swings in mood and emotion, and the extent to which they are prone to worry and focus excessively on themselves and their problems and concerns. Specifically, high emotional stability is the opposite of neuroticism, one of the central personality dimensions identified by the Five Factor Model of personality, which is the

most prominent current framework for assessing personality. By virtue of their personality, those with low emotional stability/high neuroticism are more likely than others in the same external situation to experience negative emotions and to ruminate on real or imagined problems, and are thus more likely to become burned out (Zellars, Hochwarter, Perrewé, Hoffman, & Ford, 2004).

2. *Career status*: refers to the stage one is in regarding the life of their career, whether early, mid-, or late career. Interestingly, many studies across industries suggest that early career professionals may be more at risk for burnout than their mid- and late career colleagues (Shoji et al., 2016). The reasoning provided in these studies is that early career individuals are still trying to "prove themselves" as an asset in their organization and industry. Think of junior faculty members, striving to achieve tenure and promotion in their academic careers.

3. *Marital status*: whether one is married or not. Other things equal, those who are married are at a lower risk for burnout, and this is particularly true for married men versus married women. This factor may well relate to the availability of social support in close relationships, as decades of research have consistently shown that social support is a major buffer against burnout.

4. *External locus of control*: refers to the degree to which one feels that things in their life are controlled by external forces, that is, thinking that "things just happen." Locus of control is a personality dimension that has been identified and researched for many years. Individuals with an internal locus of control feel that they can affect what happens to them. The data show that those who have an external locus of control are more likely to become burned out. These individuals are predisposed to feel and accept that they are not in control of what happens to them. One who believes – whether rightly or wrongly – that their workload is completely out of their control is unlikely to try to influence their workload, and is more likely to feel burned out. People with an external locus of control often wrongly assume constraints on their ability to influence things when those constraints do not exist. Remember that perceived control is one of the major offsets to experiencing stress, and individuals with a strong internal locus of control are predisposed by virtue of that personality trait to feel that "they can handle it" (a positive secondary appraisal).

5. *Passive coping style*: refers to responding to challenging situations by engaging in defensive efforts (e.g., distraction, avoidant behavior) rather than proactive behavior (e.g., finding a solution). For example, rather than facing the challenge of the next patient, someone with a

passive coping style might physically or emotionally withdraw from the situation.

6. *Hardiness/resilience*: the degree to which one is able to withstand challenging situations without giving up and becoming overburdened. For example, someone who does not go into "survival mode" when things get tough, but who is able to endure stress for a longer period of time. This trait is most common in those who are low in neuroticism. They do not get rattled in the face of stressful situations, and, critically, if they are stressed, they are able to bounce back quickly.

Based on this quick review of environmental/occupational and individual risk factors, we provide here a checklist (Table 1.1) for your consideration and self-reflection. The purpose of the checklist is to help you quickly identify your personal risk of susceptibility for burnout. Those with a larger number of the risk factors would be at greater risk and may unfortunately already be experiencing symptoms. However, this is by no means intended as a diagnostic tool for the purpose of officially and clinically diagnosing burnout. Rather, the hope is that those who use the checklist will gain a better understanding of their current work situation and personality and keep reading to learn about various options for helping mitigate environmental/occupational and individual risk factors. In terms of scoring, the higher the number of risk factors endorsed (i.e., "Yes") out of the twenty listed, the more at risk one is for developing burnout at work.

The focus of this chapter has been on burnout at work in general to better understand our primary focus: the burned-out physician. Many of the risk factors reported here are all too common for physicians in their work environment. The balance of the book more thoroughly investigates the work of the medical doctor and those that work with them in the healthcare delivery enterprise. The intent is to further explore the risk factors, symptoms, and outcomes in order to provide actionable solutions to help individuals, teams, organizations, and even the community and society at large deal more effectively with burnout among physicians and other healthcare providers.

The COVID-19 Effect

As we began writing this book, and continuing through the many months since, people around the world, no matter what occupation they are in, were and still are experiencing higher levels of stress and therefore greater risk of burnout as a result of the pandemic. The direct risk of catching the

Table 1.1. *Burnout risk factor checklist*

Environmental and occupational risk factors	Check yes or no
1. Low job control/autonomy	[ ] Yes [ ] No
2. High workload	[ ] Yes [ ] No
3. Excessive job demands	[ ] Yes [ ] No
4. Low social support from work colleagues	[ ] Yes [ ] No
5. Job insecurity	[ ] Yes [ ] No
6. Salary tied to billable work	[ ] Yes [ ] No
7. Work-family imbalance	[ ] Yes [ ] No
8. Unrewarding career situation	[ ] Yes [ ] No
9. High time pressure	[ ] Yes [ ] No
10. Role conflict	[ ] Yes [ ] No
11. Role ambiguity	[ ] Yes [ ] No
12. Limited physical job resources	[ ] Yes [ ] No
13. Extensively working directly with people	[ ] Yes [ ] No
14. Emotional labor required	[ ] Yes [ ] No
Individual risk factors	
1. Low emotional stability	[ ] Yes [ ] No
2. Early career status	[ ] Yes [ ] No
3. Not married	[ ] Yes [ ] No
4. External locus of control	[ ] Yes [ ] No
5. Passive coping style	[ ] Yes [ ] No
6. Low hardiness	[ ] Yes [ ] No

virus is an obvious source of stress for each and every one of us. "What if I test positive? What if a family member or coworker does?" Stay-at-home or lockdown orders (in effect widely starting in March 2020, and earlier in China and some hotspots around the globe), mask mandates, closed businesses, and now vaccination issues (what are the side effects, whether to take it, how to deal with mandates in some settings) have created stress for each and every one of us.

Likely at least one of these running monologues will feel familiar. For some, the pandemic resulted in thinking, "I can work from home (thank heaven), but I miss the social interaction. I am bored, at loose ends with nowhere to go and nothing to do." So-called essential workers, including the frontline healthcare providers, were at elevated risk. For them, the thinking went, "I can't work from home. I have to go out in the public. I am a truck driver/postal clerk/ grocery store worker." For others, it was the realization that going to work meant directly confronting the threat of infection, such an ICU nurse caring for patients who have the virus.

Still others experienced the lost jobs and businesses linked to the shutdown of economies in the United States and much of the rest of the world. Most businesses in the travel and leisure industry, for example, were and continue to be severely impacted. For workers in those industries, the monologue went like this: "I am out of work. My airline furloughed me. How will I pay my bills? My restaurant has been closed for ten weeks/four months/again after reopening for only one month. We are not going to make it." Many doctors who did not directly see COVID-19 patients saw a rapid decline in patients. "My business is down 60 percent, and I have had to furlough staff. If patients don't start coming back for routine visits, we may have to shut down." Ironically, many hospital systems have also suffered economically, leading to furloughs and layoffs even as their frontline healthcare workers were stretched to the max.

The immediate result of all the loss and uncertainty brought on by the pandemic resulted a spike in stress for everyone. John and Joe, for example, work in academic settings, and were confronted with classes transitioning to almost entirely online/remote. They had to suddenly learn new communications technologies in order to teach, and received very little training to ease the transition. Their students, too, were faced with an experience unlike the traditional college experience. Those on campus were taking classes from their dorm rooms, and were often in quarantine following a surge. College is stressful enough, but the stresses were greatly multiplied by the many drastic changes required by the pandemic.

John and Joe also consult with various business organizations, all of which have been greatly impacted by the pandemic. Some have canceled work with them out of necessity, while others have sought guidance in navigating the unprecedented and in some cases catastrophic changes to their business.

No matter what one's pre-COVID-19 level of stress was, it was dramatically increased by the crisis. Doctors, who were already identified by every survey as at high risk for burnout before, are now at even more risk.

How to Use This Book

This book is designed to accomplish three major aims. First, this chapter and Chapters 2–4 are designed to *identify the dimensions of the problem and set the stage for identifying solutions.* They are intended to inform and educate readers about burnout, what it is, what causes it, and how it looks in general but especially among physicians and other healthcare providers. These chapters also identify common burnout consequences, with particular emphasis on medical error.

Second, Chapters 5–15 are intended to *present and discuss meaningful solutions to the burnout problem for healthcare providers*. These proposed solutions cut across multiple levels, with a focus on solutions at the individual, team, organizational, and governmental/professional society levels. The main purpose for providing potential solutions across the levels that we identify is to underscore the point that efforts to mitigate burnout can and must come from multiple directions. Yes, individuals should engage in efforts to understand their own personality, become more resilient, implement strategies of self-care, and in general better manage their stress reaction (see Chapters 5 and 6). They should seek and use social support (Chapter 7), and follow the advice they freely give others about reducing their stress (Chapter 8). But in addition, teams should consider leadership and team-member strategic efforts to reduce stress (see Chapters 9 and 10) by building a positive team culture (Chapter 11). Organizations can consider work-flow changes that reduce stress (see Chapter 12); top leaders can make and advocate for changes in their organizations to resuce stress (Chapters 13 and 14); and governments and relevant governing and advisory bodies might need to look seriously at changing national healthcare policies that currently make work in healthcare increasingly stressful (see Chapter 15).

Third, Chapter 16 rounds out the book with a brief summary and a reflective call for action. We recognize that the book not only may find its way into the hands of medical professionals but also may be read by patients, family, and friends thereof. We sincerely hope that it will. Each of these folks has the potential to enact change within their sphere of influence and to lobby for change at levels beyond their immediate sphere of influence, so the major hope of Chapter 16 is to encourage individuals to engage in the reflective processes that will lead them to applying the best and most effective solutions for their situation.

Each chapter in the book concludes with a brief summary of what we are calling "key takeaways," main points we have made in each. The following are the key takeaways from this first chapter.

Key Takeaways

- While the term "burnout" is used casually in everyday conversation, burnout is actually a specific work-related syndrome, defined by the World Health Organization as "a syndrome conceptualized as resulting from chronic workplace stress that has not been successfully managed."

- Research starting in the 1970s first identified the syndrome as comprising three facets: exhaustion, cynicism, and reduced feelings of efficacy.
- The syndrome is accompanied by a range of negative, dysfunctional emotional, mental/cognitive, behavioral, and physical symptoms.
- Stress is the primary underlying factor in burnout. In the presence of a "threat," physiological and psychological reactions are automatically triggered – the fight-or-flight syndrome – to promote short-term actions to promote survival. Continuing stress can lead to burnout and a host of negative outcomes.
- Longer-term outcomes of chronic burnout include more severe versions of the personal symptoms as well as job-related negative outcomes.
- Research has consistently identified work/job-related risk factors and personal risk factors. Some jobs have characteristics that make burnout more likely. Some individuals have personality dimensions and other personal factors that predispose them to higher risk of burnout.
- This book will explain why physicians and other healthcare providers are especially at risk; explore some of the most challenging consequences of medical burnout, especially avoidable medical error; and will identify strategic "solutions" that can reduce the risk of burnout and therefore reduce the negative consequences of burnout to the physician and to their patients.
- The COVID-19 crisis, still rampant at the writing of this book, suddenly and dramatically increased the stress level, the level of fear and anxiety, and the overall level of uncertainty for everyone. Whatever the previous risk of burnout may have been for any individual, it is higher now. Physicians and other healthcare workers, already identified as at-risk in the pre-pandemic era, are now at greatly elevated risk for burnout.
- It is our hope that this book will benefit doctors and other healthcare workers, their families and friends, and their patients. We believe that it will.

REFERENCES

Ackermann, S., & Rasch, B. (2014). Differential effects of non-REM and REM sleep on memory consolidation. *Current Neurology and Neuroscience Reports*, *14*(2), 1–10.

Alessandri, G., Perinelli, E., De Longis, E., Schaufeli, W. B., Theodorou, A., Borgogni, L., … & Cinque, L. (2018). Job burnout: The contribution of emotional stability and emotional self-efficacy beliefs. *Journal of Occupational and Organizational Psychology*, *91*(4), 823–851.

Allen, J. A., Pugh, S. D., Grandey, A. A., & Groth, M. (2010). Following display rules in good or bad faith?: Customer orientation as a moderator of the display rule-emotional labor relationship. *Human Performance, 23*(2), 101–115.

Amoafo, E., Hanbali, N., Patel, A., & Singh, P. (2015). What are the significant factors associated with burnout in doctors? *Occupational Medicine, 65*(2), 117–121.

Aydemir, O., & Icelli, I. (2013). Burnout: Risk factors. In *Burnout for Experts*, ed. S. Bahrer-Kohler (pp. 119–143). Boston: Springer.

Bianchi, R., & Schonfeld, I. S. (2016). Burnout is associated with a depressive cognitive style. *Personality and Individual Differences, 100*, 1–5.

Brotheridge, C. M., & Grandey, A. A. (2002). Emotional labor and burnout: Comparing two perspectives of "people work." *Journal of Vocational Behavior, 60*(1), 17–39.

De Vente, W., Olff, M., Van Amsterdam, J. G. C., Kamphuis, J. H., & Emmelkamp, P. M. G. (2003). Physiological differences between burnout patients and healthy controls: Blood pressure, heart rate, and cortisol responses. *Occupational and Environmental Medicine, 60*(suppl. 1), i54–i61.

Ekstedt, M., Söderström, M., Åkerstedt, T., Nilsson, J., Søndergaard, H. P., & Aleksander, P. (2006). Disturbed sleep and fatigue in occupational burnout. *Scandinavian Journal of Work, Environment & Health, 32*(2), 121–131.

Erks, R., Allen, J. A., Harland, L. K., & Prange, K. (2020). Do volunteers volunteer to do more at work? The relationship between volunteering, engagement, and OCBs. *VOLUNTAS: International Journal of Voluntary and Nonprofit Organizations, 32*, 1285–1298.

Freudenberger, H. J. (1975). The staff burn-out syndrome in alternative institutions. *Psychotherapy: Theory, Research & Practice, 12*(1), 73.

Grandy, A. (2000). Understanding emotional labour: Surface acting and deep acting as predictors of burnout and effective customer service. Presented at the annual conference of the Society for Industrial and Organizational Psychology, New Orleans, LA.

ICD-11. (2019). QD85 Burn-out. Retrieved April 9, 2020, from https://icd.who .int/browse11/l-m/en#/http://id.who.int/icd/entity/129180281.

Linden, D. V. D., Keijsers, G. P., Eling, P., & Schaijk, R. V. (2005). Work stress and attentional difficulties: An initial study on burnout and cognitive failures. *Work & Stress, 19*(1), 23–36.

Maslach, C., & Jackson, S. E. (1981). The measurement of experienced burnout. *Journal of Organizational Behavior, 2*(2), 99–113.

Maslach, C., & Schaufeli, W. B. (1993). Historical and conceptual development of burnout. In *Professional Burnout: Recent Developments in Theory and Research*, ed. W. Schaufeli, C. Maslach, & T. Marek (pp. 1–16). Routledge.

Maslach, C., Schaufeli, W. B., & Leiter, M. P. (2001). Job burnout. *Annual Review of Psychology, 52*(1), 397–422.

McCarty, R. (2016). The fight-or-flight response: A cornerstone of stress research. In *Stress: Concepts, Cognition, Emotion, and Behavior*, ed. G. Fink (pp. 33–37). Cambridge, MA: Academic Press.

Montanez, R. (2021). The 7 industries where people experience burnout the fastest. Ivy Exec. Retrieved from www.ivyexec.com/career-advice/2019/the-industries-where-people-experience-burnout-the-fastest/.

Peterson, U., Demerouti, E., Bergström, G., Samuelsson, M., Åsberg, M., & Nygren, Å. (2008). Burnout and physical and mental health among Swedish healthcare workers. *Journal of Advanced Nursing, 62*(1), 84–95.

Sandström, A., Rhodin, I. N., Lundberg, M., Olsson, T., & Nyberg, L. (2005). Impaired cognitive performance in patients with chronic burnout syndrome. *Biological Psychology, 69*(3), 271–279.

Schaufeli, W. B., Bakker, A. B., & Van Rhenen, W. (2009). How changes in job demands and resources predict burnout, work engagement, and sickness absenteeism. *Journal of Organizational Behavior: The International Journal of Industrial, Occupational and Organizational Psychology and Behavior, 30*(7), 893–917.

Schaufeli, W. B., Leiter, M. P., & Maslach, C. (2009). Burnout: 35 years of research and practice. *Career Development International, 14*(3), 204–220.

Selye, H. (1950). Stress and the general adaptation syndrome. *British Medical Journal, 1*(4667), 1383.

Shoji, K., Cieslak, R., Smoktunowicz, E., Rogala, A., Benight, C. C., & Luszczynska, A. (2016). Associations between job burnout and self-efficacy: A meta-analysis. *Anxiety, Stress, & Coping, 29*(4), 367–386.

Shumski Thomas, J., Olien, J., Allen, J. A., Rogelberg, S. G., & Kello, J. (2018) Faking it for the higher-ups: Status and surface acting in workplace meetings. *Group and Organization Management, 43*(1), 72–100. doi: 10.1177/1059601116687703.

Stahl, A. (2020). 3 career paths known to cause burnout. *Forbes.* Retrieved from www.forbes.com/sites/ashleystahl/2020/07/08/3-career-paths-known-to-cause-burnout/?sh=573e77f363a4.

World Health Organization. (2019). Burn-out an "occupational phenomenon": International Classification of Diseases. Retrieved April 9, 2020, from www.who.int/mental_health/evidence/burn-out/en/.

Zellars, K. L., Hochwarter, W. A., Perrewe, P. L., Hoffman, N., & Ford, E. W. (2004). Experiencing job burnout: The roles of positive and negative traits and states. *Journal of Applied Social Psychology, 34*(5), 887–911.

CHAPTER 2

The Burned-Out Physician

All the computer-based work, record keeping, documentation and other non-clinical work is a major contributing factor. In the past, I could spend 90 percent of my time doing clinical work. Today that would be less than 50 percent.

—Physician

Burnout is a factor. The residents are especially prone to burnout. And some of them are frazzled and are abusive to the students.

—Medical student

As we discussed in the previous chapter, the work-related syndrome of burnout can be seen in a wide variety of jobs and professions. The main contributing environmental factors (such as workload and lack of control or influence over workload) that we identified appear in many work settings from food service to manufacturing to the military, from performing arts to the law to aviation, and everything in between. Let's pause for a moment and look more specifically at the workload issue, which figures so prominently in the literature and the lore on burnout.

Obviously, many of us at work are really busy, no matter our profession, and many of us don't have the level of control over our workload that we would like. Your authors and their colleagues in the academic world have joked about the "carefree life of the college professor" identified by some folks outside academia who think we are working only when we are in the classroom. In fact, John was once introduced (by a good friend with an active sense of humor) as "one of those academics who works 24/7." John thought that was surprisingly fair and accurate, contrary to the stereotype of professors. But his friend quickly elaborated. "When I say he works 24/7, you understand that as a professor that means twenty-four hours per month, seven months per year." Much good-natured laughter followed. In reality, many of us in the academy work considerably longer hours than that. A few years ago, John's institution conducted an internal survey to get staff and faculty opinions on a number of issues affecting morale. The survey asked their respondents to assess their hourly workload "in teaching, preparing for classes, grading papers and tests, advising students, conducting your own research, writing papers, chapters, or books for publication, working on departmental or college-wide committees, and other tasks." When John added up his hours for a typical week, he notched back the estimate to sixty-two hours so as not to appear too "Type A." So the question remains: Why are some of us in our various work settings, including academia, putting in fifty or sixty hours per week (or more) and yet not experiencing burnout? Workers in many professions, including the academic world, work long hours. And many have jobs that are very people-intensive to boot. But not all are at great risk for burnout. It is possible to be really busy, even as busy as a primary care doctor, and not be burned out.

In addition to the critical workload factor, in Chapter 1 we identified that some individual characteristics make people more or less prone to burnout regardless of their work situation. Of course, the highest-risk scenario for burnout is the combination of a stress-prone individual in a high-stress job.

The available data detailed in Chapter 1 clearly illustrate why medical doctors are especially at risk for burnout. We have collected interview-based data from a number of individual physicians that consistently and strongly support that assessment, and the rapidly growing research literature on physician burnout agrees. Some researchers and spokespersons identify burn-out among doctors as "more than a problem," while others use the much stronger term "crisis." John and Joe join other researchers and practitioners in thinking that "crisis" may in fact be the most appropriate word.

Note that while our discussion of burnout focuses most directly on the practicing physician, there is also a growing body of literature that suggests that others working in healthcare are similarly at risk. Later in this chapter we will turn our attention to physicians' assistants, nurses, pharmacists, and other healthcare workers. We will briefly review current relevant published data on these other healthcare providers, and we have also included epigraphs from several of these healthcare providers based on our interviews with them. All are at risk. But for now, let's focus first and foremost on the physician.

Why Are Doctors at Risk?

Let's look at the career of the medical doctor, starting with the good news. Years of rigorous training and evaluation are required in order to become a physician. John and Joe have both worked with many undergraduate students who were aiming for medical school and a career as a doctor, and we have witnessed the reality of pre-medical students in college. Not only do they have to have very good grades in even the most challenging hard science courses, but they must score well on the standardized admissions test for medical school, the MCAT, and they have to secure positive recommendations from their on-campus pre-medical committee. They are an extremely select group, with cognitive abilities and motivation level well above average. To get into medical school they must compete successfully with a cohort composed of others with similar ability and drive. During their four years of medical school, they discover it is common for most (or all) of their fellow med students to have been in the top 10 percent of their undergraduate class. If they are successful, their training continues further in a residency for an additional three to five years.

Doctors emerge from their many years of training as medical experts and practitioners in one of the most highly admired and respected professions in the world. In a recent reputable international survey, "medical doctor" was identified as the number one most respected profession in the world among fourteen other professions that require higher education and high professional qualifications (Shukla, 2019). Nurses came in as the sixth most respected profession in this survey, barely behind police officer and head/senior teacher. A different survey conducted by Gallup identified the most trusted, honest, and ethical professions. On this US-based survey, medical doctors came in third, behind nurses at number one, and slightly ahead of pharmacists (Reinhart, 2021). Many similar surveys always include doctors and other healthcare professionals as high on the list of respected professions.

Doctors should never have to wonder whether their work makes a difference. They care for the sick, they cure patients. Some do life-saving surgeries. On classical scales in organizational science research that rate "job enrichment" (Hackman & Oldham, 1976) and measure underlying facets of the job such as skill variety (developing and using a range of skills), task identity (seeing whole pieces of work to completion), task significance (meaningfulness, value), autonomy (ability to "do it your way"), and feedback (from the work and from others, knowing how well you are doing), the work of the medical doctor should score very high (with the possible exception of the autonomy facet, as we will explain).

Doctors are also positioned to earn a very nice living. Depending on their specialty, their material rewards can be substantial indeed, comparable to those of other highly trained professionals, and on a par with the psychic rewards they reap for caring for the sick and afflicted. That's the good news.

On the other hand, the medical profession has changed gradually over the last few decades, and even more dramatically in recent years. Indeed, the first three environmental/occupational risk factors identified in Table 1.1 in Chapter 1 (i.e., low autonomy/control, excessive demands, and workload) have become increasingly prevalent for doctors, offsetting some of the "job enrichment" inherent in the medical career. One critical example is how the rise of electronic health records (EHR) has increased workload and negatively impacted the amount of time that a doctor spends per patient. In the Physicians Foundation survey (a major nationwide survey), the nearly 9,000 responding doctors estimated that they spent an average of 23 percent of their time with such record keeping (Physicians Foundation, 2018). A separate, direct observational study of emergency department doctors showed that their self-report estimate might be dramatically low – by half! Physicians were observed to spend a whopping 44 percent of their time on data entry compared to 28 percent of their time spent in direct patient care (Hill, Sears, & Melanson, 2013).

This shift from patient time to paperwork time has had a notable effect on job satisfaction among physicians. In the Physicians Foundation survey, 79 percent of respondents identified the most satisfying element of their medical practice as "patient/physician relationships." A wide range of factors were identified as "least satisfying," including "EHR design/interoperability," "regulatory/insurance requirements," and "loss of clinical autonomy" (Physicians Foundation, 2018). Those job-related negatives represent time away from the primary source of physicians' job satisfaction: quality time with patients.

Various other compliance requirements further restrict clinical time and add to the overall workload of the medical doctor. Doctors and other healthcare experts whom we interviewed as part of our research for this book consistently decried the "numbers game" they were in as a result of the prevailing volume-based/fee-for-service model (see environmental/occupational risk factor #6). This factor dictates that doctors' income commonly depends on the number of patients they see, rather than some measure of the quality of the work they do. While there are some developing efforts to link compensation and bonuses to quality metrics, many such attempts to date have proven cumbersome and difficult to manage, and are not yet widespread.

Many doctors have enormous patient rosters. The average number of patients seen per day by respondents in the 2018 Physicians Foundation survey was 20.2, with a small percentage seeing "61 or more" per day (Physicians Foundation, 2018). Around 80 percent of those survey respondents indicated they are at full capacity or are overextended. Clearly, many doctors are experiencing crushing workload along with reduced clinical time and reduced autonomy.

Compared to decades ago, an increasing and surprising number of doctors at all stages of their career report deep disappointment and pessimism about the state of things in medical practice. Indeed, more than half of those surveyed (55.3 percent) described their professional morale and their feelings about the current state of the medical profession as "somewhat negative" or "very negative." Only 7 percent responded "very positive." Questions about the future state of the profession and whether the respondent would recommend medicine as a career for their children or other young people yielded similar negative responses (49 percent responding negatively). For example, 27.4 percent said that if they personally had the chance to choose medicine again, they would not (Physicians Foundation, 2018). The vast majority want to be doctors. They want the career of service they envisioned and trained for. They want to make it work. They want to reduce the risk of burnout.

As more and more practitioners are feeling more stress and less joy, a number of physicians self-report that they are directly experiencing the symptoms of burnout. Nearly 80 percent of the Physicians Foundation survey respondents report feeling the symptoms of burnout at least sometimes, with a good number of those indicating they "always" feel burned not (Physicians Foundation, 2018). Other surveys (such as the Medscape 2019 report and those mentioned in Chapter 1) find similar results.

Note that in most cases, female physicians report higher levels of burnout than their male counterparts (Physicians Foundation, 2018). The speculation is that women are not only in general more likely to self-report burnout and to seek treatment; they may also experience more challenges in achieving reasonable work-life balance, given the primary role that women usually play in caring for children and managing the household. Much research shows that professional women with families still bear the brunt of routine household responsibilities. For these and no doubt many other reasons, female physicians may not "just" overreport, compared to their male peers; they may indeed be at significantly greater risk for burnout.

What Symptoms Are Common in the Burned-Out Physician?

There's a crucial point to emphasize right up front. Stress is cumulative, not compartmentalized. Whatever the source, it adds up. We don't have separate internal "buckets" for work stress, home stress, financial stress, aging stress, health stress, traffic stress, and so on. It all "goes into the same place." The stress reaction, the general adaptation syndrome, does not differentiate or respond differently to different types of stressors. If the primary appraisal says, "It's a threat to me" and the secondary appraisal says, "I am not sure I can cope," the same stress reaction is triggered whether the stressor is an argument at home, a traffic accident on the way to work, or the hurry to finish with this patient and see the next one who has been waiting for an hour.

While doctors are rightly respected, even revered, for the work they do, they are also human beings, with all the joys and challenges that everyone else faces. They are likely to have a spouse or partner. They may also have children or aging parents who need care, or have school-age or college-age children who need their active support. They will have a mortgage or monthly rent obligation as well as other bills. They may have student loans (which, in their case, can be very large indeed). They commute to work. They may have a demanding boss and conflicts at times with coworkers. In short, they have all the potential stressors that nonmedical people do, in addition to the distinctive stresses of their career as outlined above.

Doctors are prone to experience all the stress-related symptoms experienced by nonmedical employees, and then some. They are prone to feel fatigued, run down, and exhausted. They may have physical symptoms such as the dreaded sleep disruption, headaches, upset stomach, and muscle tension, which may range from mild and intermittent to chronic. They may express their frustration in angry outbursts, leading their relationships at home and at work to suffer. They may find it hard to concentrate and may make more mistakes at work and outside work.

These symptoms, markers of burnout laid out in some detail in Chapter 1, are common to people working inside and outside medical practice. They are not unique to medical doctors. But – and this is a key "but" – for medical doctors, the nature of their work and their level of professional responsibility make burnout more likely for them, and make their burnout symptoms more dangerous to others as well as to themselves.

How are doctors' symptoms dangerous to others? The short answer is that their stress-to-the-point-of-burnout endangers their patients. A central focus of this book is patient safety, as impacted by the connection between burnout and medical error.

The Burned-Out Physician and Medical Error

As we have noted earlier, burnout puts anyone suffering from the syndrome at greater risk for making errors. The physical and emotional exhaustion associated with the syndrome make it harder than usual to concentrate, and therefore more likely than usual to forget a key task, miss a step, or do the wrong thing. A factory worker may mix raw ingredients incorrectly, resulting in a bad batch of product. A sales representative may forget a promised follow-up meeting with a potential client, costing a potential sale. An HR professional may file an employee's performance review in the wrong folder or inadvertently release confidential information. Such errors are of course problematic, whenever or wherever they happen, and burnout makes them more likely.

But some professionals, prominently including doctors, are in a different category in terms of the potential impact of their errors. Errors in the operating room (OR), emergency room (ER), or intensive care unit (ICU) can yield serious, even catastrophic outcomes for patients. In a large-scale national survey, a surprising percentage of doctors (14 percent in a recent national survey) acknowledge that their mental/emotional state associated with burnout and depression makes them more likely to commit errors (Clark, 2021; Kane, 2019). As visible as the issue is with teams in the OR, ER, or ICU, other physicians, including primary care doctors, are also at risk. So are nurses, physicians' assistants, pharmacists, and indeed any professionals in the chain of medical care.

Let's turn our attention for a moment to those other healthcare workers.

Burnout in Nurses, Physicians' Assistants, Pharmacists, and Other Healthcare Providers

As much as our central focus is on the medical doctor, we can't ignore the others who also play crucial roles in the overall healthcare delivery process. During our interviews, we were struck by the similarity and consistency of the responses from different healthcare professionals. While the workspace and role of a nurse, pharmacist, medical student, lab technician, and physician obviously differ, all of our interview subjects were in effect describing the same stresses. They all acknowledged burnout from their own experience, and while they used their own terms to describe what they had seen and what they had experienced, the ways they described it were remarkably similar. If we edited out comments that were job-specific (e.g., supporting a doctor, filling prescriptions, prepping for exams, labeling blood draws) it would be hard to guess which comments were from a medical student, pharmacist, lab tech, or any of the other healthcare professionals we interviewed.

In the chain of events and interactions that involve the treatment of a patient (e.g., when a patient gets a diagnosis, receives treatment, is prescribed medication, gets that medication from a pharmacist, perhaps undergoes surgery, is hospitalized, receives additional medications, is cared for by nurses, and is released), any professional can make a mistake. And again, burnout puts any individual in a higher risk category for making mistakes, including mistakes that can seriously harm a patient.

Nurses have recently come into focus as a group facing very similar pressures as those faced by physicians. The self-reported burnout data among nurses are broadly comparable to those seen among physicians (Sutherland, 2017). According to this survey of nurses, nearly half of the 600 nurses surveyed in the United States indicated that they were considering leaving the profession. The most common reasons given were burnout-related, including feeling overworked (the most common reason, given by 27 percent of the respondents), followed by just not enjoying the job anymore, and time spent on nonclinical requirements of excessive paperwork/EHRs. Recent studies have identified certain nursing specializations as especially burnout-prone, that is, oncology, emergency, and long-term care (Gaines, 2019).

While the causal chain may be difficult to unravel, it is interesting that medical facilities in which nurses report higher levels of burnout also have the highest levels of patient infections unrelated to their primary medical issue (surgical site infections and urinary tract infections; Cimiotti, Aiken, Sloane, & Wu, 2012). While such correlational data do not allow us to draw causal conclusions, it is at least possible (and probably most likely) that burnout is the culprit, leading to more avoidable errors committed by nurses.

The developing body of research on pharmacists and burnout points to startlingly similar conclusions. While fewer studies by far have been conducted with pharmacists (at least to date), those that have researched them have found, if anything, higher levels of self-reported burnout among pharmacists than among physicians and nurses. Data gathered in 2017 and 2018 showed that as many as 64 percent of 193 responding pharmacists reported feeling burned out, showing at least one of the three major defining symptom categories (emotional exhaustion, depersonalization, and diminished effectiveness; Traynor, 2019). In a larger study with 974 responding pharmacists, the self-reported burnout percentage was 61 percent (Jones, Roe, Louden, & Tubbs, 2017). The reasons identified by respondents to these surveys will sound quite familiar, namely, heavy workload and low control. These results are actually more intense than reported levels of burnout in physicians and critical care nurses.

We will turn in the next chapter to the question of what specific kinds of medical errors are most likely to occur. However, before leaving the general topic of the impacts of burnout on healthcare providers, there is another especially crucial and painful issue to be addressed. We noted earlier that burnout puts doctors at risk, not only for committing avoidable errors that can be harmful to and even fatal for their patients but also for harming themselves as well. In addition to possible overuse of alcohol or other drugs, surprisingly common among physicians, doctors are at greater risk for suicide than those in other professions.

Suicide in the Healthcare Professions: The Ultimate Negative Effect of Burnout

The suicide rate among doctors is commonly reported to be between two and three times the national average (Anderson, 2018; Gerada, 2018). Reliable research sources indicate that one doctor dies by their own hand every day in the United States, totaling as many as 400 per year according to the most current estimates (Clark, 2021). Suicide is much more common among male doctors than female doctors, but then there are many more male than female doctors. Correcting for representation in the profession by gender, the suicide rates are about the same (Anderson, 2018).

Depression is obviously a correlate and predictor of suicidal thoughts and actions. The vast number of individuals who attempt suicide, successfully or not, are suffering from depressive disorder. Current data show that the estimated/self-reported rate of depression among physicians is about the same as in the general population, which may seem surprising, given the high correlation between burnout (which we know to be high) and depression (Anderson, 2018). However, doctors may be much less likely to acknowledge their depression and seek help for it for a variety of reasons. Recent statistics suggest that 40 percent of physicians are reluctant to seek mental health treatment (Dyrbye et al., 2017), and only 6 percent of female physicians willingly disclose when they have been diagnosed with a mental health condition (Gold, Andrew, Goldman, & Schwenk, 2016). They may fear losing hospital privileges, or even their license by appearing to need mental health care. Even if trusted, confidential care is available, they may not feel they have the time to pursue it, given their workload. Relatively prone to substance abuse as a result of burnout anyway, doctors have more access than others to lethal substances (poisoning or overdosing are prominent techniques among doctors who commit suicide, especially among female doctors; Anderson, 2018).

Clearly, medical doctors are at risk for suffering the ultimate devastating effect of burnout. To the extent we can get meaningful data, the risk to others in the healthcare chain appears to be comparable. As we have suggested based on the research summarized so far, nurses, pharmacists, physicians' assistants, and other healthcare professionals face many of the same workload issues as doctors, report similar levels of burnout, and are at comparable risk for any of the consequences of burnout, including, sadly, suicide (Androus, 2020; Barker, 2018; Brusie 2019; Firth, 2019; King & Bradley, 2019; Rizzo, 2018).

Let's look for a moment more specifically at nurses. The existing suicide data for nurses are similar to the data for physicians, though there are challenges in getting accurate numbers, as there has been less focus on nurses than on doctors. Quoting a recent study by Rizzo (2018):

> A general internet search produced no public data identifying a national nurse suicide rate in the United States, yet data on suicide rates are readily available for physicians, teachers, police officers, firefighters, and military personnel. The Centers for Disease Control and Prevention (CDC) maintains a restricted National Violent Death Reporting System (NVDRS), which is the most comprehensive death registry by suicide coded by occupation. It has been growing yearly, with data available for 40 states, the District of Columbia, and Puerto Rico. The dataset has not been queried for nurse suicide statistics.

Insofar as we do have data to allow us to draw conclusions for nurses of any gender, we can see that their suicide rates are significantly higher than the rates for males and females in the general population (Firth, 2019). Much as with nurses, the data for pharmacists and physicians assistants are closely similar, though those data are also very sparse and limited, and apples-to-apples comparisons are difficult to make.

A Global Issue

While our focus thus far has been on healthcare workers in the United States, the problems highlighted here in terms of burnout, error, and even suicide are by no means unique to healthcare practice in that country. Studies conducted in the United Kingdom, Canada, China, France, Spain, Portugal, Germany, and many other parts of the developed or developing world show the same patterns as those seen in the United States (Locke, 2019; "Physician burnout," 2019).

Consider the data collected from 968 physicians in the United Kingdom in 2018 (Locke, 2018). This survey found that 30–40 percent of UK doctors self-reported feeling burnout, especially general practitioners (GPs). A total of 64 percent of respondents reported being depressed "because of the job." Remember the close association between burnout and depression. The responding physicians' depression was associated with being less motivated to be careful (16 percent), more likely to make error they would not ordinarily make (14 percent), and even making a serious error that would harm a patient (3 percent). A total of 25 percent said their symptoms were so severe that they were thinking of leaving medical practice, and 66 percent said that the duration of their symptoms lasted at least one to more than two years. The reasons for burnout were closely similar to the reasons given by US-based physicians in comparable surveys; for example, 47 percent said their main concern was "too many bureaucratic tasks." Only 10 percent were currently in treatment or planning to seek treatment for burnout and depression (but 11 percent checked "prefer not to answer"). Of those experiencing burnout, 53 percent said they plan to retire early, and 37 percent were thinking of leaving medicine for a different career. Overall, about one third report being somewhat to very unhappy with their work life. In terms of coping strategies, 42 percent isolate themselves, 41 percent talk it out, and 40 percent exercise, but 30 percent eat junk food, 30 percent drink alcohol, and 26 percent binge eat. In this UK study, 80 percent of the respondents work solely in the National Health Service, and another 11 percent in both the NHS and private practice. Only 19 percent of the respondents were GPs, but again they were especially prone to report symptoms of burnout.

A similar UK study with a smaller group of respondents ($N = 417$) found that 55 percent of respondents met the criteria for burnout. Interestingly, these studies focus considerable attention on GPs and the pressures of their role (Cook, 2019). The British Medical Association estimated recently that as many of 90 percent of GPs may face a high risk of burnout. A further study reported in *The Guardian* includes data from a survey of 1,651 doctors in all specialties across all of the United Kingdom. The data, published in the *BMJ Open* journal, indicate that nearly a third of UK doctors may be suffering from high levels of burnout, stress, and "compassion fatigue," and identify a primary cause as "excessive workloads in the NHS" (Campbell, 2020). It appears that accident and emergency (A&E) doctors and GPs are the most likely to report feeling burned out (Campbell, 2020).

Regarding suicide data, as one recent article stated,

> Throughout time and across the world, doctors have always had higher rates of suicide compared with the general population and with other

professional groups. Female doctors in particular have higher rates – 2.5–4.0 times the rate by some estimates. The reasons for suicide among doctors – as in the general population – are often related to un- (or under-) treated depression, bipolar disorder, or substance misuse. (Gerada, 2018)

With the arguable exception of bipolar disorder, the other suicide correlates are also correlates of burnout.

While it is beyond the scope of this book, in our research we have noted a growing crisis in China in the number of attacks by the public on doctors and other healthcare providers. To an extent greater than that experienced in the United States, doctors, nurses, and other healthcare workers in China have the additional stress of risk of physical attack and even death at the hands of disgruntled patients or their family members (Physician, 2019).

Reliable data from low median-income countries are hard to come by, but there is no reason to expect that the incidence of the burnout crisis is any less severe. Indeed, there is good reason to suspect that the problem may be greater there, as healthcare providers in the developing world are likely to experience heightened levels of environmental/job-related risk factors (workload, lack of adequate tools and other resources, etc.).

Summing up, physicians and other healthcare workers are facing unprecedented and increasing levels of stress that can lead to burnout. Burnout exacts a toll – sometimes severe and even life-threatening – on the sufferer. Given that the work of the medical professional so strongly impacts others, their increased likelihood of error puts those they have sworn to help at greater risk of harm. Burnout, for so many reasons, is a global crisis in healthcare.

The COVID-19 Effect

It is obvious from our comments in earlier parts of this book that the pandemic is dramatically increasing the workload and intensity of the work of frontline healthcare providers. The usual lag between data collection and data publication in refereed journals means that reliable scientific research on the mid-crisis current state is sparse so far, but growing rapidly. Much of the data available to us online consists of opinion pieces by practitioners and other medical experts, which are informed opinions to be sure, but based on scant data. But as those opinion pieces and the few rigorous studies trickle and then flood in, they will no doubt uniformly support the position that the crisis is fueling physician burnout to a phenomenal degree.

As their workloads spiked, doctors and nurses alike found themselves working long hours and experiencing more severe cases and more fatalities than ever before. It is fair to call them soldiers-in-combat. They were personally at risk due to their exposure to sick patients, and many of them were largely or entirely cut off from their friends and families in order to protect them. In fact, somewhere between 80,000 and 180,000 health and care workers have died from COVID-19 from January 2020 to May 2021 (WHO, 2021). "Second" and "third waves" became a fact of life in many parts of the world, including the United States, which reeled during the Delta and Omicron surges of cases. Even as vaccination rates rise, burnout risk for frontline healthcare providers remains at an all-time high.

While we may not automatically think of pharmacists as being on the front line, the reality is that their workload had been dramatically increased by the pandemic too. As soon as widespread COVID testing became available, pharmacists began providing such services. COVID testing was just another addition to the other factors that had been gradually increasing their workload and reducing their autonomy prior to the pandemic, but it also increased the people-intensity of their work and their potential exposure to the virus even as it reduced the time they could devote to their primary role of filling prescriptions carefully and accurately.

When the crisis slows to a close, many of these frontline healthcare workers will experience depression, anxiety, and even some form of post-traumatic stress disorder (PTSD). They will need the help and support of mental health resources. Much has been written about the mental health crisis for the population at large as a result of lockdowns, economic disruption, disruption in school schedules, fear of catching and spreading the virus, and on and on. The front line is experiencing all of that too! Researchers are warning of a strain on mental health services, as so many of us are experiencing unprecedented levels of stress. So it is with the front line. A challenge, though, is doctors' reluctance to acknowledge their burnout symptoms and seek professional help. For a variety of reasons, they are more prone to "go it alone."

Doctors who are not on the battlefield are also experiencing substantially heightened stress in addition to their preexisting levels of stress. Before the pandemic, their work-related challenges have been mostly related to workload, that is, the burden of nonclinical administrative activities, lessened autonomy, and other factors we have explored in our book so far. Now the challenge is maintaining their practice in light of the precipitous drop-off in patients related to COVID-19. Their challenge is to survive the current state and prepare for the post-crisis "next normal" even as their risk of burnout is at an all-time high.

Key Takeaways

- It is widely acknowledged that burnout among doctors and other healthcare providers is more than a problem; it is a crisis of epic proportions.
- As a group, doctors are intelligent, talented, hard-working achievers who are dedicated to healing. Theirs is a highly respected profession. On the face of it, they should be no more at risk for burnout than anyone who has a job, a mortgage, a spouse or partner, routine daily challenges, and so on.
- Medical practice has changed dramatically in recent years, such that workloads have increased and autonomy has decreased, which in combination are a formula for increased stress. A major result of systems changes impacting medical practice is that physicians have less and less clinical time with their patients, and more time spent on administrative tasks.
- A surprisingly large percentage of physicians report symptoms of burnout, generally low morale, and pessimism about the current and future state of medical practice.
- Burnout among physicians not only manifests in the wide range of psychological and physical symptoms that are markers of the syndrome; burned-out physicians are more likely to commit errors, which in some cases can have devastating consequences.
- Surveys taken among other healthcare providers, such as nurses and pharmacists, show closely similar results to surveys taken among practicing physicians. Burnout is a growing crisis among all who are in the chain of healthcare delivery.
- Suicide might be seen as the ultimate negative effect of burnout. While suicide can occur for other reasons, burnout is identified as a major reason among doctors, where the suicide rate is several times that of the general public.
- Suicide rates among other healthcare providers are similarly elevated, and burnout is widely acknowledged as a major contributing cause.
- While much of the research we draw on was conducted in the United States, the burnout problem is by no means limited to that country. Comparable studies conducted in the United Kingdom show the same patterns as seen in the US data, with the additional emphasis on the

role of the general practitioner as a healthcare "gatekeeper" with the additional stresses that designation brings.

- The COVID-19 pandemic has suddenly and dramatically increased the stress level, and thus the risk of burnout, both among frontline workers and among private practices that faced loss of their business.

REFERENCES

Anderson, P. (2018, May 8). Doctors' suicide rate highest of any profession. WebMD. Retrieved from www.webmd.com/mental-health/news/20180508/doctors-suicide-rate-highest-of-any-profession#1.

Androus, A. B. (2020, December 15). Nurse suicides: Unveiling the shrouds of silence. Registered Nursing.org. Retrieved March 2, 2021, from www.registerednursing.org/articles/nurse-suicides/.

Barker, A. (2018). Pharmacist suicide risk: What we know and don't know. The Happy PharmD. Retrieved from www.thehappypharmd.com/pharmacist-suicide-risk-what-we-know-and-dont-know/.

Brusie, C. (2019). Study reveals alarming statistics on nurse burnout. Nurse.org. Retrieved from https://nurse.org/articles/nurse-burnout-statistics/.

Campbell, D. (2020). Third of UK doctors report burnout and compassion fatigue. *The Guardian*. Retrieved September 28, 2020, from www.theguardian.com/society/2020/jan/27/third-of-uk-doctors-report-burnout-and-compassion-fatigue.

Christianson, M. K., Sutcliffe, K. M., Miller, M. A., & Iwashyna, T. J. (2011). Becoming a high reliability organization. *Critical Care, 15*(6), 314. doi: 10.1186/cc10360.

Cimiotti, J. P., Aiken, L. H., Sloane, D. M., & Wu, E. S. (2012). Nurse staffing, burnout, and health care–associated infection. *American Journal of Infection Control, 40*(6), 486–490.

Clark, M. (2021). 50+ shocking physician burnout statistics you'll never believe. *Etactics*. Retrieved from https://etactics.com/blog/physician-burnout-statistics.

Cook, J. (2019). Majority of UK doctors are burnt out, study shows. *GP Magazine*. Retrieved September 28, 2020, from www.gponline.com/majority-uk-doctors-burnt-out-study-shows/article/1584800.

Dyrbye, L. N., West, C. P., Sinsky, C. A., Goeders, L. E., Satele, D. V., & Shanafelt, T. D. (2017). Medical licensure questions and physician reluctance to seek care for mental health conditions. *Mayo Clinic Proceedings, 92*(10), 1486–1493. https://doi.org/10.1016/j.mayocp.2017.06.020.

Firth, S. (2019). Suicide risk in nurses higher than general population. MedpageToday. Retrieved from www.medpagetoday.com/nursing/nursing/81003.

Gaines, K. (2019). Joint Commission tackles nurse burnout in new report. Nurse.org. Retrieved from https://nurse.org/articles/joint-commission-tackles-nurse-burnout/.

Gerada, C. (2018). Doctors and suicide. *British Journal of General Practice, 68* (669), 168–169.

Gold, K. J., Andrew, L. B., Goldman, E. B., & Schwenk, T. L. (2016). "I would never want to have a mental health diagnosis on my record": A survey of female physicians on mental health diagnosis, treatment, and reporting. *General Hospital Psychiatry, 43*, 51–57. https://doi.org/10.1016/10.1016/j .genhosppsych.2016.09.004.

Hackman, J. R., & Oldham, G. R. (1976). Motivation through the design of work: Test of a theory. *Organizational Behavior and Human Performance, 16* (2), 250–279.

Hill, R. G., Jr., Sears, L. M., & Melanson, S. W. (2013). 4000 clicks: A productivity analysis of electronic medical records in a community hospital ED. *The American Journal of Emergency Medicine, 31*(11), 1591–1594.

Jones, G. M., Roe, N. A., Louden, L., & Tubbs, C. R. (2017). Factors associated with burnout among US hospital clinical pharmacy practitioners: Results of a nationwide pilot survey. *Hospital Pharmacy, 52*(11), 742–751. https://doi .org/10.1177/0018578717732339.

Kane, L. (2019). Medscape National Physician Burnout, Depression & Suicide Report 2019. Medscape. Retrieved from www.medscape.com/slideshow/ 2019-lifestyle-burnout-depression-6011056#2.

King, C., & Bradley, L. A. (2019). Trends & implications with nursing engagement. PRC Custom Research. Retrieved from https://prccustomresearch .com/wp-content/uploads/2019/PRC_Nursing_Engagement_Report/PRC-NurseReport-Final-031819-Secure.pdf.

Locke, T. (2018). Medscape UK Doctors' Burnout & Lifestyle Survey 2018. Medscape. Retrieved from www.medscape.com/slideshow/uk-burnout-report-6011058#:~:text=Burnout%20continues%20to%20be%20a,to% 20be%20most%20at%20risk.

(2019). Medscape global physicians' burnout and lifestyle comparisons. Medscape. Retrieved from www.medscape.com/slideshow/2019-global-burn out-comparison-6011180#5.

Physician burnout: A global crisis. (2019). *The Lancet, 394*(10192), 93. doi: https://doi.org/10.1016/S0140-6736(19)31573-9.

Physicians Foundation. (2018). 2018 Survey of America's Physicians Practice Patterns & Perspectives. Retrieved from https://physiciansfoundation.org/ wp-content/uploads/2018/09/physicians-survey-results-final-2018.pdf.

Reinhart, R. (2021, January 14). Nurses continue to rate highest in honesty, ethics. Gallup. Retrieved March 2, 2021, from https://news.gallup.com/poll/ 274673/nurses-continue-rate-highest-honesty-ethics.aspx.

Rizzo, L. H. (2018). Suicide among nurses: What we don't know might hurt us. American Nurse. Retrieved from www.myamericannurse.com/suicide-among-nurses-might-hurt-us/.

Shukla, V. (2019). Top 10 most respected professions in the world. Value Walk. Retrieved from www.valuewalk.com/2019/03/top-10-most-respected-profes sions/.

Sutherland, S. (2017). Survey finds nearly half of nurses considering leaving the profession. RN Network. Retrieved from https://rnnetwork.com/blog/rnnet work-nurse-survey/.

Traynor, K. (2019, January 31). Pharmacists examine risks, remedies for burnout. ASHP.org. Retrieved March 2, 2021, from www.ashp.org/news/2019/01/30/ pharmacists-examine-risks-remedies-for-burnout?loginreturnUrl=SSOCheckOnly.

World Health Organization (WHO). (2021). Health and care worker deaths during COVID-19. Retrieved from www.who.int/news/item/20-10-2021- health-and-care-worker-deaths-during-covid-19.

CHAPTER 3

Types of Medical Error

I am at the front end. If I miss something, that mistake can send us down the wrong path. Initial diagnosis is crucial.

—Primary care physician

I think about burnout more now than I did before. There's no time to double check, and no one to check after me. The pace is too quick. It's like a "prescription assembly line"! I'm afraid an overworked colleague will make a mistake that kills someone.

—Pharmacist

We know that burnout is a surprisingly common workplace syndrome, with specific, well-identified symptoms. We also know that doctors and other healthcare professionals are particularly at risk for experiencing burnout and that one of the prominent consequences of burnout is error. Error can have devastating effects on patients and further add to the level of stress that the healthcare provider is experiencing. On that latter point, there is a phenomenon identified in some of the practice literature as the "second victim effect." The first victim is the patient who was harmed by an avoidable error, while the second victim is the medical professional who becomes aware that they made the mistake that resulted in harm to the patient. The "second victim" experiences additional stress, in a kind of vicious cycle.

Let's explore the kinds of errors that can occur in healthcare, and then see how and where they occur in the chain of events from initial diagnosis to treatment and beyond. First, though, let's put healthcare work in a broader context by examining the concept of the "high reliability organization" and how healthcare fits clearly into that category.

High Reliability Organizations and Error Control

Research in the broad area of occupational safety and health has identified a specific class of "industries" where error management is especially critical since the consequences of error can be so profound. Such organizations are identified collectively as high reliability organizations (HROs; Christianson, Sutcliffe, Miller, & Iwashyna, 2011). While this term can be defined in a variety of ways, all HROs have a critically important common denominator: since error can have far-reaching and devastating effects on both the worker who makes the mistake and on others impacted by the mistake, error control is therefore mission critical. An additional defining characteristic of HROs is that the nature of the work is extremely complex. Operators require years of training, a high level of certification/licensing, and frequent retraining. Whatever the specific nature of the work of an HRO is, "it has to be done right every time." High reliability means reliable, safe, and error-free (to the extent humanly possible) performance and outcomes.

Both Joe and John have had the opportunity to conduct research and to consult extensively with a number of HROs, including companies in the nuclear industry. Uncorrected mistakes within the nuclear industry can – as history has shown –lead to disastrous consequences for thousands of people. While safety has always been a prime concern in the nuclear industry for this reason, the industry became especially sensitive to error and error management in the wake of the Three Mile Island incident in 1979 (Backgrounder, 2018). While employees at that nuclear power plant were ultimately successful at interrupting and containing the near-meltdown that occurred at Unit 2 at Three Mile Island (TMI-2), analyses after the fact concluded that a delay of only a few more hours would have resulted in a potentially catastrophic event not unlike the Chernobyl accident in the Ukraine in 1986, where an explosion and fire resulted in massive amounts of radioactive material actually being released into the atmosphere. Due to the greatly different design of US nuclear facilities, which surrounded the reactor with containment buildings, the likelihood of such a massive, life-threatening release into the atmosphere from the TMI-2 incident was extremely low. But a total meltdown of the nuclear core could have contaminated groundwater and had other environmentally devastating effects. Studies of both of these high-profile incidents in the nuclear industry reveal a common pattern of errors that can compound to the point of triggering a serious event.

In response to these events and the potential of similar future disasters, the nuclear industry has long identified error management as essential to safe operation. Industry leaders have incorporated training in a variety of specific, best-practice techniques of communication and coordination that include double-checking and triple-checking directions and responses, the use of multiple backup safety systems, and training employees to respond promptly and effectively to error when it does occur. If an error is made, nuclear operators are trained to work together as a cohesive unit to promptly identify, isolate, correct, and ultimately learn from it. Such safety/error-management training is incorporated into initial licensing classes for nuclear control room operators (managed by the Nuclear Regulatory Commission), and is reinforced continually in ongoing refresher training in the simulator, managed by the utilities (Frye, Harrington, & Kello, 1987; US NCR, 2020). In one company with which we have worked, continual training for licensed nuclear control room operators is seen as so important that literally one week out of every five is spent in the classroom and the simulator refreshing on operational issues, especially on error control.

We have also worked intensively with the commercial aviation industry, another HRO focused intensively on error management. While domestic air travel is extremely safe in full-size aircraft, accidents in past years have severely challenged several airline companies. Following a massive fire and catastrophic crash of one of ValuJet's planes in 1996, the company had to take drastic public relations measures to help shake the flying public's association of the carrier with the fatal crash, and ValuJet ultimately chose to change the company name to AirTran. Not surprisingly, the investigation into this accident by the National Transportation Safety Board identified a chain of uncorrected errors as the cause of this catastrophic accident. In this particular case, it was not the "usual" pilot error, but rather a series of mistakes involving the storage of hazardous combustible materials in the cargo hold of the plane that led to the fire and the fatal crash (National Transportation Safety Board, 1997). Air carrier manufacturers also experience the need for safe operations, including the need to avoid the risk to their reputation that error-driven accidents can cause. For example, the recent Boeing 737 Max 8 accidents have greatly disturbed the public's perception of the manufacturer's commitment to safety and transparency in acknowledging (and not hiding) mistakes (Gelles, 2019). Safe operation is obviously essential to the success of manufacturers as well as carriers in aviation, and safe operation at any level means error management and error reduction.

We have had a firsthand glimpse into how things can go wrong in the cockpit. During work at the University of Texas with one of the best aviation research teams in the world, John had the opportunity to listen to dozens of cockpit voice recordings from accidents that had occurred around the world over a period of many years. It quickly became apparent that human error is the culprit when things go wrong in the cockpit. This finding is supported by a number of historical accident scenarios that confirm that there is virtually always a chain of human errors leading to a given catastrophic outcome. Like the nuclear industry, aviation has designed training and operations protocols to decrease the possibility of error and to promote the capturing and correcting of error if it does occur. Cockpit teams (usually a two-person team, comprising captain and first officer), assisted by air traffic control, flight attendants, and other team resources, are also trained to communicate and coordinate their activities in order to make fewer errors. These teams are also more likely to quickly identify, isolate, and correct any errors that do occur, therefore intervening early in the chain of events that could lead to an accident.

The medical operating room team can obviously be viewed as closely similar to a flight crew or a nuclear control room team: The surgeon is the captain of the team, or the "senior operator" in charge, and the surgeon works in close proximity to the anesthesiologist. These doctors are assisted by nurses who are typically involved in every aspect of preoperative preparation, the surgery itself, and postoperative care. A safe and effective surgical team must establish a clear plan of action beforehand, continually communicate and coordinate their activities during surgery, identify and respond adaptively to changing conditions, check and verify assumptions throughout their procedure, and in general ensure that all members of the team are on the same page at all times (Healey, Undre, & Vincent, 2006). Their patient, their patient's health, and even the patient's life depends on "doing it right" and without errors. If error does occur, the team must swiftly identify it, isolate and correct it, and learn from it.

Around the same time that the early research in the HROs of aviation and nuclear operations was being established in the 1980s and 1990s, it became apparent to researchers that the OR shared many of the features with the cockpit and the control room (Parush, 2007). As a result, training programs similar to those in aviation (called "crew resource management" training, or CRM) and nuclear operations (sometimes called "team and diagnostics training") have taken place in many medical training settings (Helmreich, Wilhelm, Kello, Taggart, & Butler, 1990; Pizzi, Goldfarb, & Nash, 2001). In aviation and nuclear operations, these training programs are aimed squarely at error reduction, and CRM-type training for medical students is as well. Such training programs are not mandated but are increasingly common, and have been found to increase students' awareness of the risk and consequences of error (e.g., Kutaimy et al., 2018). Interestingly, such programs have a similar trajectory to early aviation CRM programs, in that such programs are not mandated, at least not yet, and they focus on increasing awareness and positive attitude, and the behaviors that promote coordinated actions of the team. Later evolutions of CRM programs in aviation showed that the increased awareness and positive attitude on the part of pilots were reflected in the more effective use of the behavioral tools and techniques of crew coordination, and overall in safer behavior during actual operations. We would expect the same from early introduction and subsequent reinforcement of patient-safety initiatives in healthcare.

Beyond the introduction of error-reduction safety principles in early training, healthcare systems in general are increasingly embracing core principles of the HRO, with excellent results. A study published in May 2019 reviewed efforts by the US Veterans Administration (VA) to evaluate strategies for implementing HRO practices in the VA (Veazie, Peterson, & Bourne, 2019). The authors of this review article examined twenty published studies of HRO implementation in healthcare settings and found that the "most commonly reported implementation strategies . . . were: (1) developing leadership, (2) supporting a culture of safety, (3) building and using data systems to track progress, (4) providing training and learning opportunities for providers and staff, and (5) implementing interventions to address specific patient safety issues." In evaluating the effects of implementation of such HRO strategies, seven published studies reported reductions ranging from 55 to 100 percent in "serious safety events" after implementation of relatively comprehensive HRO strategies. Those data are comparable to those seen when explicit HRO methodology is introduced in other industries, and are obviously very encouraging for the healthcare enterprise.

Burnout in Nuclear Operations and Aviation

Burnout is not, at least of this writing, identified as a primary concern (much less a crisis) in the nuclear industry, certainly not to the extent that it is in healthcare. There is essentially no literature – research-based or popular – on the risk of burnout leading to major errors in the nuclear industry. Studies on incidents such as TMI-2 have attributed the error-riddled event not mainly to stress-based or burnout-related factors, but mainly to equipment design flaws, inadequate training, and – critically – poor communication and coordination among the team of operators, all of which resulted in a chain of errors. If there is a burnout concern in the nuclear industry, it might be that the work of the nuclear control room operator is so routinized and "managed by the technology" that boredom and thus loss of vigilance and situational awareness can be an issue. Anecdotally, we have observed that nuclear operators have been known to joke that their job is "babysitting the technology." The systems run on autopilot until there is an off-normal condition requiring all hands on deck. But the design of typical biocompatible shift schedules to minimize sleep disruption or "shift lag" as well as the promotion of individual- and team-based communication and coordination strategies help to minimize the likelihood of both overwork-related and potential boredom-related burnout, and thus the likelihood of error (Frye, Harrington, & Kello, 1987; US NCR, 2020). As with domestic commercial aviation in the United States, the nuclear industry has a remarkable history of remarkably safe operation.

In the past there was little to no literature on potential burnout among airline pilots, but that appears to be undergoing a change. In a recent large sample of airline pilots, 40 percent of the responding pilots indicated they experience burnout regularly (Demerouti, Veldhuis, Coombes, & Hunter, 2019). That is a surprising outcome indeed, and one that has received nowhere near the level of attention and concern that burnout among doctors has. The results with the pilot sample indicate that increasing job demands appear to be the main culprit. Evidence of fatigue and burnout-related performance loss appears most readily during simulator training, which pilots are required to undergo on a regular basis. Pilots' performance in the simulator was worse in terms of overall flight success and attention to detail (hence, performance loss) among those who indicated they experience burnout regularly. Still, there is nothing in the aviation literature that we have found that comes close to the medical literature in terms of the frequency and prevalence of burnout, and the risks associated with burnout, including the risk of a major error in actual operations. And it is worth noting that the traditional focus in the simulator has been assessing the individual pilots' technical skills. This may be changing to some extent, but in our direct experience the simulator has not encouraged the use of the skills that are taught in CRM classes, which focus not only on individual awareness but also on communication and coordination among members of the team to catch errors before they compound into an accident. It is noteworthy that, despite the developing concern about burnout among pilots, there has not been a fatal crash involving a major US-based carrier in more than ten years as of this writing. Compare that with the estimated number of 250,000 medical error–related fatalities annually in the United States!

At the end of this chapter we look at the COVID effect as it impacts healthcare workers. We might briefly note here that airline personnel, prominently including pilots, are severely affected by the pandemic as well. As of this writing, commercial airlines in the United States and abroad are experiencing a financial crisis of epic proportions. Many pilots (and other airline employees) have been furloughed or laid off, and as the industry continues to struggle, there is likelihood that the cuts will be deeper and will last longer. The very recent imposition of vaccine mandates by some carriers is likely to result in at least some further reductions in staff, namely, those who choose not to take the shot. There are indications that, as of this writing, that is already happening. Some industry experts are speculating that it may be five to ten years before the airline industry recovers to anything near 2019 levels. That devastating level of uncertainty must surely add to the stress level of pilots, even those who are still employed.

We will further explore the issue of burnout in medical care in relation to errors shortly. First, however, we know that in any HRO work environment, adverse outcomes are most often the end result of a series of mistakes rather than a single, sudden, large-scale event. Let's begin by exploring this aptly named framework: the "chain of events."

The Chain of Events

Research on HROs going as far back as the 1970s identified that most accidents by far were the end result of a chain of events – or, more accurately, were composed of a chain of errors that could have been anticipated and avoided, or at least isolated and mitigated at any of several of the links in the chain. Most accidents resulted from multiple causes, such as a combination of systems failures, teamwork failures, and/or individual failures. Major accidents are sometimes characterized as "the perfect storm." In our extensive experience as safety researchers and consultants, most accidents show the same pattern: a concatenation of events, often in themselves relatively minor, which could be easily addressed. At any point in the chain of events, the individual errors could be preempted or interrupted. However, without identification and correction, errors can and do compound and lead to more serious consequences.

People are naturally prone to fear the "sudden, large-break event" more than they fear (or even consider) the series of minor flubs or missed opportunities that can add up to result in an accident. For example, those individuals with a morbid fear of flying are more likely to picture engines exploding than they are to picture pilot and copilot not communicating needed information effectively and making a series of mistakes as a result of lack of coordinated teamwork. It is true that a sudden large break can occur (however, if you trace back through a root cause analysis, you usually find systems deficiencies that made the large break effectively inevitable sooner or later). But the sudden large break, whatever its roots, is the dramatic exception, not the rule. Most accidents, whether mild or catastrophic, have multiple causes and are the result of the error chain.

Consider the following real-life situation (albeit a mild one!) that happened to John, to illustrate how the common chain-of-events accident pattern develops.

John: "When traveling and staying in a hotel, I always park my own rental car. But at one particular hotel downtown in a major city, valet parking was the only option. Upon arrival I turned over my car to a valet, and got my claim ticket. All was well until the morning of my flight back home. I had been told the previous evening to call down fifteen to twenty minutes before I needed my car to give the extra-busy valets time to retrieve it, as the hotel was fully booked and many people would need their cars around the same time in the morning. Shortly before I finished packing, I accordingly called down and gave my name and ticket number. When I got down to the lobby with bags in hand, I noticed that other hotel guests were stepping directly into their waiting cars. While at first I assumed they had called ahead, before I did, I then saw several guests come down with claim tickets in hand, and wait only a few minutes before their cars arrived. This happened again and again, and I began to feel uneasy.

"About twenty minutes into this drama, I asked a valet about my car and showed him my claim. He looked in vain through a cabinet containing a large rack overflowing with car keys and claim ticket stubs at his station. He assured me that meant another valet must be bringing it around now, so it should arrive momentarily. More time went by. I repeated the process with another valet, who also could not find my keys. 'We have a black one,' he offered tentatively, gesturing toward it, 'could that be yours?' It was not. I was pretty sure mine was silver. The minutes ticked by, and the departure time of my flight was approaching rapidly.

"Finally, the desk clerk came out. 'The gentleman who has your car,' he explained, 'is at the airport. He just called in and said he should be back here to get his car and give you yours in about thirty minutes.' Sure enough, thirty minutes later, the other fellow returned, and I was able to get in my own actual rental car, drive to the airport, and board the plane just in time, all the while wondering how an impossible event like this could actually happen. Talk about the perfect storm!

"Let's analyze this comedy of errors. The other fellow must have called down earlier than I. Somehow, they brought him my car. Did they not double check the ticket? Did he not realize it was not his car? (I remembered the one valet offering me someone else's car.) It turned out that the other fellow's rental car was identical to mine. He was also about my size. Neither he nor I needed to adjust the seat or mirrors. The settings were perfect for both of us. What an unlikely chain of events!

"How could this comedy of errors have been prevented? If I could have parked my own car, which I always do when allowed, there would have been no issue. If the valet had checked the other man's ticket correctly, the valet could have given him his car and not mine. No issue. If the man was not my size, surely he would have noticed right away that the settings were not right, and that this was not his car. Problem avoided."

John tells this true story because it illustrates how accidents actually occur. A system is flawed . . . or an effective system is violated . . . people don't double-check their information at critical junctures . . . they are in a rush . . . they don't communicate and coordinate with others . . . off-normal conditions occur . . . and at the end of a chain of unlikely events, things go wrong. The accident occurs. They are not the sudden, large-break, single-cause events that people fear. They are the end result of a series of errors, each error in itself often very minor.

Having reviewed dozens and dozens of accidents, from minor OSHA recordables, lost time accidents, and fatalities in industrial settings to major catastrophes such as airline crashes, nuclear incidents, offshore oil rig explosions, and chemical releases, we can assure you that the chain of events model is clearly in effect in the vast majority of such accidents. And it is just as likely to happen in healthcare as it is on a plane, in a nuclear control room, or in any other work setting.

So, we know that in HROs, error must be controlled. Let's turn our attention from the general category of HRO to the healthcare delivery process specifically. How much of a problem is medical error?

Medical Error: How Big Is the Problem?

The short answer is: very big. The longer answer can vary, as it is difficult to obtain complete and accurate data. Estimates from the late 1990s gave a figure of an estimated 98,000 deaths per year in the United States attributable to avoidable medical error (Kohn, Corrigan, & Donaldson, 2000; Pham et al., 2012). Subsequent estimates were dramatically higher, ranging between 210,000 and 440,000 deaths per year (Carver & Hipskind,

2019; Mallory, Weller, Bloch, & Maze, 2013). Based on the latter estimates, medical error is now widely identified as the third leading cause of
death in the United States. Though the most recent estimates at just over
250,000 are obviously much lower than the 440,000 figure, research
conducted at the Johns Hopkins Medical School supports the "third
leading cause" claim, suggesting that 9.5 percent of annual deaths in the
United States are medical error–related (Johns Hopkins Medicine, 2016).
That is an astonishing figure. Read it again: 9.5 percent of all deaths each
year in the United States.

It is crucial to understand what kinds of errors most commonly occur,
and where, how, and why such errors occur. Of course, it is at least equally
important, and arguably more important, to identify strategies that effectively reduce the frequency of harmful and potentially lethal medical errors
by reducing the burnout that is so often a major contributing cause of such
errors. But first, let's look at what the data show in terms of the types of
errors that commonly occur.

What Kinds of Errors Occur in Healthcare?

Within healthcare delivery, patients are most likely to encounter errors of
planning and/or errors of execution, and errors of commission and/or
errors of omission. These classes of errors can occur anywhere in the chain
of events that constitute healthcare services. Later we will turn to the
question of "where." But first we will occupy ourselves with "what kinds"
of errors.

According to the widely used classification proposed by the Institute of
Medicine, the primary medical error categories are as listed in Table 3.1
(Kohn, Corrigan, & Donaldson, 2000).

Let's examine these categories in more detail, focusing first on diagnostic errors.

Diagnostic Errors

A 2016 report found that diagnostic errors (planning) were the primary
source of errors in emergency departments (Carver, Gupta, & Hipskind,
2021). The most frequently misdiagnosed conditions found in this report
of some 332 patient-injury claims included "acute cerebral vascular accident, myocardial infarction, spinal epidural abscess, pulmonary embolism,
necrotizing fasciitis, meningitis, testicular torsion, subarachnoid hemor-
rhage, septicemia, lung cancer, fractures, and appendicitis." Commonly

Table 3.1. *Types of medical errors*

Category	Item	Example
Diagnostic errors	• Error or delay in diagnosis • Failure to employ indicated tests • Use of outmoded tests or therapy • Failure to act on results of monitoring or testing	• When a patient having a heart attack is told their pain is from acid indigestion • Not ordering an MRI or incorporating test results into treatment • Using an older version of a screening questionnaire • Failure to review all medical records and test outcomes
Treatment errors	• Error in performance of an operation, procedure, or test • Error in administering treatment • Error in the dose or method of using a drug • Avoidable delay in treatment or in responding to an abnormal test • Inappropriate care	• Wrong patient's blood was used for an osteoporosis test • Removing a healthy kidney instead of the cancerous one • Physician does not provide complete instructions for use of medication • Communication of test results is through mail rather than phone call or email • Applying cardiac procedures to a healthy patient
Preventive errors	• Failure to provide prophylactic treatment • Inadequate monitoring or follow-up of treatment	• Patient not given appropriate vaccinations • Poor handoffs at the end of an employee's shift
Other errors	• Failure of communication • Equipment failure • Other system failure	• Lack of coordination • Stent failure leading to heart attack • Restrictive appointment types (set for only one condition when patients have multiple conditions)

identified causes included failure to order appropriate tests (omission) and failure to accurately interpret abnormal test results (commission). Also identified were communication/coordination errors, including failure of all to review the medical records, and lack of coordination, especially among the medical team. Another 2001 study in an emergency and accident department found 953 diagnostic errors in 934 patients, with the most common error being missed fractures, typically due either to failure to accurately read a radiograph or failure to order radiography in the first place (Guly, 2001).

A similar study of emergency department errors over a two-year period (2013–2015) in England and Wales found results in line with the

US-based studies cited above (Hussain et al., 2019). Quoting from the abstract of the study:

> There were 2288 cases of confirmed diagnostic error: 1973 (86%) delayed and 315 (14%) wrong diagnoses. One in seven incidents were reported to have severe harm or death. Fractures were the most common condition (44%), with cervical-spine and neck of femur the most frequent types. Other common conditions included myocardial infarctions (7%) and intracranial bleeds (6%). Incidents involving both delayed and wrong diagnoses were associated with insufficient assessment, misinterpretation of diagnostic investigations and failure to order investigations. Contributory factors were predominantly human factors, including staff mistakes, healthcare professionals' inadequate skillset or knowledge and not following protocols.

However, medical errors are certainly not limited to emergency departments nor to the diagnostic phase. But keep in mind that an uncorrected error at the outset, in initial diagnosis, will compound as the subsequent steps unfold. A flawed diagnosis, if not corrected, will lead to inappropriate treatment. Let's look next at the more common types of treatment errors.

Treatment Errors

Once a diagnosis is made, treatment is then provided by physicians, nurses, pharmacists, and other healthcare providers. Errors in this broad, multistep category of treatment might, for example, include a mistake during a surgical operation, such as a wrong-site surgery. This dreadful category of error can obviously have catastrophic consequences. The general category of surgical error also typically includes the subtypes of wrong procedure (something was done that the patient didn't need) and wrong patient (a procedure intended for another was applied to the patient; PS Net, 2019). While rare, such surgical errors do occur in the operating room as well as in other settings (e.g., ambulatory surgery). And given the large number of such procedures that are performed every day, a tiny percentage of such a huge number is still a significant number. Again, the consequences of removing a healthy kidney instead of the cancerous one, or applying cardiac procedures to a patient who has a healthy heart (or failing to apply such procedures to the patient who needs them) can be extraordinarily severe.

Treatment errors also might involve incorrectly administering a test, administering the wrong test, or failure to respond in a timely way (if at all) to a positive test. For example, Joe regularly has a lipid panel test performed to check his cholesterol. The communication of the results happens in any of several ways, including sometimes in the office at a follow-up visit, sometimes via a phone -call from the physician or another medical professional, and sometimes in a letter in the mail. On one occasion, the letter in the mail came, and Joe found out both his lipid results and the puzzling announcement that he did *not* have osteoporosis. Upon follow-up with the healthcare provider, Joe discovered that evidently his blood was used for both his lipid panel and for a test of osteoporosis intended for another patient's blood draw.

Other treatment errors can involve medications, a treatment chain in which many healthcare providers play a part (Tariq, Vashisht, Sinha, & Scherbak, 2021). Consider a "typical" hospitalized patient. The physician prescribes medications at specified dosages, with directions as to how and when the drugs are to be administered. The drug has to be the right medication in the right amount, delivered to the right patient of course, and the directions have to be correct. To avoid adverse drug interactions, other medications the patient might be taking have to be taken into account. The pharmacist has to correctly read and fill the prescription for the patient. Nurses have to accurately follow the medication protocol to ensure that the correct patient is receiving the correct dosage of the right drug at the right time. A mistake in any of those links can result in adverse, even fatal, consequences.

More General Errors: Preventive and Other

As noted earlier, a 2016 study found that there were relatively common communication/coordination errors, including failure of all to review the medical records and lack of coordination/poor handoffs, especially among all members of the medical team (Carver, Gupta, & Hipskind, 2021). We will have much more to say about sources of error that are not solely, or even mainly, attributable to individual mistakes, but rather involve teamwork, or systems failures.

How about post-treatment care, including careful patient follow-up and monitoring? Even if diagnosis and treatment have been error-free (or any errors have been caught and corrected), there is always the chance that the patient will have postoperative problems. These problems might include an unanticipated drug allergy or some other adverse event that could have been avoided through careful monitoring and detailed follow-up. For example, hospital-acquired infections and pressure sores are not uncommon among hospitalized patients, either postop or preop.

According to the National Institutes of Health (NIH), a medical error is a "preventable cause of an adverse effect of medical care, even when the result is not harmful to the patient" (Carver, Gupta, & Hipskind, 2021). Obviously, the impact of the error is greater when the adverse effect is in fact harmful to the patient, and greater still of course when the result is an avoidable fatality. From their data, the NIH further identifies commonly occurring errors as comprising "adverse drug events and improper trans-fusions, misdiagnosis, under and over treatment, surgical injuries and wrong-site surgery, suicides, restraint-related injuries or death, falls, burns, pressure ulcers, and mistaken patient identities." NIH also notes that errors are more likely to happen in high-pressure situations (ICUs, ORs, EDs) and during complex procedures or when caring for high-risk patients (Zavala, Day, Plummer, & Bamford-Wade, 2018). An elderly cancer patient experiencing heart failure is more likely to encounter a medical error than a fit twenty-year-old presenting with a simple fracture.

Other sources identify errors that occur at a relatively frequent rate, including medication errors, errors related to anesthesia, hospital-acquired infections, missed or delayed diagnosis, avoidable delay in treatment, inadequate follow-up after treatment, inadequate monitoring after a pro-cedure, failure to act on test results, failure to take proper precautions, and technical medical errors (Carrie, 2021). However, still another source lists the nine most common medical errors as follows: "adverse drug events, catheter-associated urinary tract infection (CAUTI), central line-associated bloodstream infection (CLABSI), injury from falls and immobility, obstetrical adverse events, pressure ulcers, surgical site infections (SSI), venous thrombosis (blood clots), and ventilator-associated pneumonia (VAP)" (Carver, Gupta, & Hipskind, 2021).

While medication errors and errors in diagnosis are mentioned promi-nently in most studies, there appears at this point to be no definitive listing of *the* most common types of errors. The delivery of healthcare is a complex, multistep process, with many links in the "chain," and so many error types are possible in any phase of the treatment process and in a wide variety of medical settings. However, the vast number of studies conducted in all HROs suggest that uncorrected errors in the earliest phases of a scenario would be the most crucial. Errors in the diagnostic phase deter-mine the course of treatment from that point on and inform later errors. While other errors may occur down the chain, the initial uncorrected error sets the course.

John once had the unpleasant experience of what was later correctly diagnosed as acid reflux. When he experienced its symptoms for the first

time, he went to a local emergency treatment facility. Upon initial exam-
ination, the doctor and nurse quickly began initiated procedures for
addressing a cardiac event. John's wife, a retired nurse who knew John
had no history of cardiovascular problems, questioned this approach. The
examining nurse explained that John's unusually high heart rate and chest
"pain" informed their course of action. However, what the medical team
did not realize was that John had used a high-powered twelve-hour nasal
spray an hour or so earlier, to ease allergy-related nasal congestion. He
didn't think to mention it, and no one asked. Once that came to light, the
course of treatment shifted dramatically to be quicker, simpler, much less
unpleasant, and ultimately successful.

The pressure on the first point of contact – in other ones, the first to
diagnose and the "gatekeeper" for subsequent treatment – may be a central
reason that emergency department staff, primary care physicians (in the
United States), and general practitioners (in the United Kingdom) are
universally identified as being at such elevated risk for burnout. Their
diagnosis sets the stage for every aspect of treatment that follows. Their
errors can impact the effectiveness and safety of the treatment the patient
receives from them or others in the chain of events.

It is critical for physicians and other healthcare professionals to be aware
of the most common types of errors and how and where such errors occur
in the chain of events aiming to support patient care and promote patient
well-being. Figure 3.1 illustrates how critical the initial diagnosis is, in this
case on the part of ER doctors.

A Note on Nurses, Burnout, and Medication Errors

A recent survey of almost 1,800 nurses in the United States found that
more than half of the respondents self-reported physical and mental health
concerns related to burnout (Melnyk et al., 2018). More than half of those
experiencing burnout symptoms reported that they had made medical
errors in the past five-year period, and a significant portion of those are
likely medication errors, as nurses are the point of contact for dispensing
medication to hospitalized patients. Medication errors can vary widely in
type, ranging from errors in ordering (e.g., failure to order, ordering at the
wrong time, ordering an incorrect or unauthorized drug), errors in preparation, and errors in administration (e.g., the incorrect route of administration, giving the drug to the wrong patient, extra dose, or wrong rate;
Tariq, Vashisht, Sinha, & Scherbak, 2021). Other medication errors can
be categorized as errors in monitoring (failure to account for patient liver

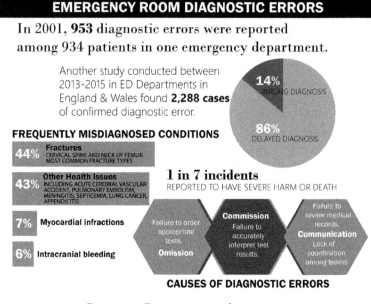

EMERGENCY ROOM DIAGNOSTIC ERRORS

In 2001, **953** diagnostic errors were reported among 934 patients in one emergency department.

Another study conducted between 2013-2015 in ED Departments in England & Wales found **2,288 cases** of confirmed diagnostic error.

14% WRONG DIAGNOSIS

86% DELAYED DIAGNOSIS

FREQUENTLY MISDIAGNOSED CONDITIONS

44% Fractures
CERVICAL SPINE AND NECK OF FEMUR MOST COMMON FRACTURE TYPES

43% Other Health Issues
INCLUDING ACUTE CEREBRAL VASCULAR ACCIDENT, PULMONARY EMBOLISM, MENINGITIS, SEPTICEMIA, LUNG CANCER, APPENDICITIS

7% Myocardial infractions

6% Intracranial bleeding

1 in 7 incidents
REPORTED TO HAVE SEVERE HARM OR DEATH

Commission
Failure to accurately interpret test results.

Omission
Failure to order appropriate tests.

Failure to review medical records.

Communication
Lack of coordination among teams

CAUSES OF DIAGNOSTIC ERRORS

Figure 3.1 Emergency room diagnostic errors.

and renal function, failure to document allergy or potential for drug interaction) and compliance (not following protocol or rules established for dispensing and prescribing medications; Tariq, Vashisht, Sinha, & Scherbak, 2021). In addition to these error types, we must mention the possibility of mislabeling tissue samples for biopsy, that is, assigning samples to the wrong patient.

Recent data suggest that medication errors are most common at the ordering or prescribing stage (Elden & Ismail, 2016). Ordering errors, including the healthcare provider writing the wrong medication, wrong route or dose, or the wrong frequency, account for almost 50 percent of all medication errors. Between 30 and 70 percent of the time, medication errors are caught and addressed by nurses and pharmacists (Tariq, Vashisht, Sinha, & Scherbak, 2021), placing additional burden on staff.

Significant mortality, morbidity, and economic loss have been linked to medication errors. An estimated 7,000–9,000 deaths in the United States annually are caused by medication error. It is likely that multiples of that number of people experience nonfatal adverse reactions related to a pre-scribed medication. Furthermore, the costs of treating medication-related errors alone are estimated to exceed $40 billion each year (Tariq, Vashisht, Sinha, & Scherbak, 2021).

These errors fall upon the attending physician, the pharmacist, and the nurse, and potentially to the lab technician, to varying degrees. But the critical issue is not "Who is to blame?" but how to intercept and correct errors before they can compound into a serious adverse event. When prescribing and delivering medication, physicians and nurses experiencing burnout are more prone to making mistakes along the way due to their reduced cognitive and physical resources. All healthcare workers should strive to understand the kinds of errors that are especially likely in their duties, and to identify those that are especially problematic in their practice in order to maintain a high level of vigilance at every step in the treatment process.

The COVID-19 Effect

The pressures leading to preexisting levels of avoidable medical error have compounded under the circumstances of the pandemic. The long hours, heavy workload, and traumatic experiences of many frontline healthcare providers make medical error more likely (Hay-David et al., 2020; Tejos et al., 2020). Many doctors were confronted with wearing multiple layers of personal protective equipment (PPE) such as masks and face shields, some of which was unfamiliar and much of which was uncomfortable. In addition, these layers of PPE impacted the effectiveness of communication, even when working in familiar teams. Others found themselves working outside the areas in which they were trained or where they normally practice.

New faces may contribute to the risk of medical errors. As the need for doctors and nurses spiked, some have come out of retirement to help. Conversely, some medical and nursing students had their graduations accelerated, enabling them to practice early. In some parts of the United States, medical school graduates who passed their Step 1 and Step 2 exams but had not been placed in a residency (so-called assistant physicians, or APs) were allowed to practice in some circumstances (Frellick, 2020). Medical "teams" comprised members who did not ordinarily work together, thus lacking key rapport and knowledge essential to effective teamwork. For these and many other reasons, burnout risk has and continues to be at a recent high – likely an all-time high – as is the likelihood of mistakes.

A related phenomenon is beginning to show up in the burnout literature during the pandemic: the "burnout domino effect" (Roulet, 2020).

This effect refers to the observation that individuals who are experiencing burnout affect coworkers in the same way. Their depressed mood can be in itself contagious, thus adding to the general level of burnout at their workplace. Similarly, if a burned-out coworker drops out, their workload will most likely be absorbed by others, adding additional stress. So, my burnout not only can affect your mental state negatively, but if it causes me to quit, my departure can add further to your workload. The burnout of one person can increase the risk of burnout in others and, of course, the associated risk of making mistakes.

As of now, there are no data of which we are aware on whether the crisis has shifted the locus or typology of medical error in any significant way. For COVID-19 patients, enhanced testing has made it likely that positive cases will be correctly diagnosed. Errors are more likely than before, we would speculate, in the treatment phase, for reasons outlined above, though at present we have seen no widespread data to that effect.

But there are developing studies that suggest that medication errors involving nurses may be increasing disproportionately. In what is being called "pandemic nursing care," rushed and overworked nurses who are seeing unprecedented numbers of critically ill patients are now more likely to make a major medication error (PSQH, 2020). Medication errors may be significantly underreported due to the increased pace of work and the fear of retribution (Morrison, Cope, & Murray, 2018; Shaw, 2012). One ICU nurse who was interviewed describes a perfect storm for serious medication errors in the ICU:

- The hectic pace and disorganization of pandemic nursing
- The constantly underresourced healthcare environment
- High nurse-to-patient ratios due to staffing shortages
- The exhausting and continual donning of PPE
- The criticality of patients who require multiple high-alert medication infusions
- The stashes of medication infusions located in patients' drawers and closets
- The inability for timely response to smart pump alarms
- The need for any available nurse, not necessarily the assigned nurse who is familiar with the patient, to manage critical infusions.

Most of the nurse-involved medication errors identified in this interview occurred after retrieving the wrong concentration of an infusion from stashes that were left in patients' rooms by nurses on earlier shifts. This was described as follows: "Multiple concentrations of a drug may be available for one patient in response to required fluid restrictions due to renal and/or heart failure. Programming errors, titration errors, and mix-ups among the numerous infusions also occurred frequently." There are also tragic cases in which a smart pump was incorrectly programmed, such that intended infusions of norepinephrine were actually infusions of fentanyl that resulted in a fatality. For non-COVID-19 patients, there are no obvious reasons to think that the locus of errors would be altered by the pandemic, at least as of this writing.

Key Takeaways

- Healthcare is an example of a high reliability organization (HRO) in which error can have catastrophic consequences and must be controlled.
- Burnout is identified as more of a problem in healthcare than in other HROs, though there are developing trends in aviation.
- Most accidents are the end result of a chain of events, not a sudden "large break" event. Errors, if they are not identified and corrected, can compound to the point that an accident occurs. Many of the errors are, in and of themselves minor mistakes. Again, the chain-of-events pattern is seen in most accidents.
- Medical errors are of several main types: diagnostic, treatment, preventive, and "other."
- Diagnostic errors are relatively common, especially in emergency departments. Obviously, a missed or incorrect diagnosis will have ripple effects into the treatment phase and beyond.
- Medication errors are relatively common treatment errors, and can have serious negative consequences for the patient. Nurses are disproportionately more likely to be involved in all types of medication error. "Wrong site surgery" is a much rarer but similar error type with potentially devastating consequences.
- More general errors can include mistakes in the postoperative phase of healthcare delivery.
- Errors are more likely to occur in critical, high-pressure situations, such as intensive care units, operating rooms, and emergency departments, especially when doctors and other healthcare providers are conducting complex procedures and/or when caring for high-risk patients.
- While medication and diagnostic errors are widely reported as most common, errors can occur in any phase of healthcare delivery.

- The COVID-19 pandemic has dramatically increased the stress level of healthcare providers. As of this writing, there are no studies to suggest that the pandemic has shifted the locus of medical errors in any significant way. However, recent studies indicate that medication errors made by nurses in ICUs during the pandemic do appear to be on the rise. The main effect of the pandemic to date, though, is to dramatically increase the risk of error of any and all types in the chain of healthcare delivery.

REFERENCES

Carrie, Anne. (2021, March 16). The 8 most common root causes of medical errors. Always Culture. Retrieved March 5, 2021, from https://alwaysculture .com/hcahps/communication-medications/8-most-common-causes-of-medi cal-errors/.
Backgrounder. (2018). Three Mile Island accident. US NRC. www.nrc.gov/docs/ ML0402/ML040280573.pdf.
Carver, N., & Hipskind, J. E. (2019). *Medical Error.* Treasure Island, FL: StatPearls.
Carver, N., Gupta, V., & Hipskind, J. E. (2021). *Medical Error.* StatPearls (online). Treasure Island, FL: StatPearls Publishing.
Christianson, M. K., Sutcliffe, K. M., Miller, M. A., & Iwashyna, T. J. (2011). Becoming a high reliability organization. *Critical Care, 15*(6), 314. doi: 10 .1186/cc10360.
Demerouti, E., Veldhuis, W., Coombes, C., & Hunter, R. (2019). Burnout among pilots: Psychosocial factors related to happiness and performance at simulator training. *Ergonomics, 62*(2), 233–245. doi: 10.1080/00140139 .2018.1464667.
Elden, N. M., & Ismail, A. (2016). The importance of medication errors report-ing in improving the quality of clinical care services. *Global Journal of Health Science, 8*(8), 54510. https://doi.org/10.5539/gjhs.v8n8p243.
Frellick, M. (2020). Assistant physicians: COVID-19 draws notice to new type of physician. Medscape. Retrieved from www.medscape.com/viewarticle/933312? nlid=136210_5402&src=wnl_dne_200703_mscpedit&uac=321353MK&impID= 2445421&faf=1.
Frye, S., Harrington, D., & Kello, J. (1987). Teaching teamwork in the control room: A systematic approach. *The Nuclear Professional, 2*(2), 21–24.
Gelles, D. (2019, October 28). Boeing 737 Max: What's happened after the 2 deadly crashes. *New York Times.* www.nytimes.com/interactive/2019/busi ness/boeing-737-crashes.html.
Guly, H. R. (2001). Diagnostic errors in an accident and emergency department. *Emergency Medicine Journal: EMJ, 18*(4), 263–269. doi: 10.1136/emj.18.4.263.
Hay-David, A. G. C., Herron, J. B. T., Gilling, P., Miller, A., & Brennan, P. A. (2020). Reducing medical error during a pandemic. *The British Journal of*

Oral & Maxillofacial Surgery, 58(5), 581–584. doi: 10.1016/j.bjoms.2020.04.003.

Healey, A. N., Undre, S., & Vincent, C. A. (2006). Defining the technical skills of teamwork in surgery. *Quality & Safety in Health Care, 15*(4), 231–234. doi: 10.1136/qshc.2005.017517.

Helmreich, R., Wilhelm, J., Kello, J., Taggart, W., & Butler, R. (1990). Reinforcing and evaluating crew resource management: Evaluator/LOS instructor reference manual. NASA/University of Texas at Austin.

Johns Hopkins Medicine. (2016). Study suggests medical errors now third leading cause of death in the US. Retrieved on April 30, 2019, from www.hopkinsmedicine.org/news/media/releases/study_suggests_medical_errors_now_thir d_leading_cause_of_death_in_the_us.

Hussain, F., Cooper, A., Carson-Stevens, A., Donaldson, L., Hibbert, P., Hughes, T., & Edwards, A. (2019). Diagnostic error in the emergency department: Learning from national patient safety incident report analysis. *BMC Emergency Medicine, 19*(1), 77. doi: 10.1186/s12873-019-0289-3.

Kohn, L. T., Corrigan, J., & Donaldson, M. S. (2000). *To Err Is Human: Building a Safer Health System*, vol. 6. Washington, DC: National Academies Press.

Kutaimy, R., Zhang, L., Blok, D., Kelly, R., Kovacevic, N., Levoska, M., Gadivemula, R., & Levine, D. (2018). Integrating patient safety education into early medical education utilizing cadaver, sponges, and an inter-professional team. *BMC Medical Education, 18*(1), 215. https://doi.org/10.1186/s12909-018-1325-9.

Mallory, S., Weller, J., Bloch, M., & Maze, M. (2013). The individual, the system, and medical error. *British Journal of Anaesthesia 3*(6), 179–182. doi: 10.1093/bjacepd/mkg179.

Melnyk, B. M., Orsolini, L., Tan, A., Arslanian-Engoren, C., Melkus, G. D. E., Dunbar-Jacob, J., . . . & Braun, L. T. (2018). A national study links nurses' physical and mental health to medical errors and perceived worksite wellness. *Journal of Occupational and Environmental Medicine, 60*(2), 126–131.

Morrison, M., Cope, V., & Murray, M. (2018). The underreporting of medication errors: A retrospective and comparative root cause analysis in an acute mental health unit over a 3-year period. *International Journal of Mental Health Nursing, 27*(6), 1719–1728. doi: 10.1111/inm.12475.

National Transportation Safety Board. (1997). In-flight fire and impact with terrain Valujet Airlines flight 592 DC-9-32, N904VJ. www.ntsb.gov/investigations/Pages/DCA96MA054.aspx.

Parush, A. (2007). Safety in medical operating room and aviation: Common issues. HCI News and Ideas from the Human Oriented Technology Lab. *Hot Topics, 6.*

Pham, J. C., Aswani, M. S., Rosen, M., Lee, H., Huddle, M., Weeks, K., & Pronovost, P. J. (2012). Reducing medical errors and adverse events. *Annual Review of Medicine, 63*, 447–463. https://doi.org/10.1146/annurev-med-061410-121352.

Pizzi, L., Goldfarb, N. I., & Nash, D. B. (2001). Crew resource management and its applications in medicine. In *Making Health Care Safer: A Critical Analysis of Patient Safety Practices*, ed. A. J. Markowitz (pp. 511–519). Rockville, MD: AHRQ Publications.

PS Net. (2019, September 7). Wrong-site, wrong-procedure, and wrong-patient surgery. PS Net. Retrieved from https://psnet.ahrq.gov/primer/wrong-site-wrong-procedure-and-wrong-patient-surgery.

PSQH. (2020, September 11). During the pandemic, aspire to identify and prevent medication errors and to avoid blaming attitudes. Health Leaders Media. Retrieved from www.healthleadersmedia.com/nursing/during-pandemic-aspire-identify-and-prevent-medication-errors-and-avoid-blaming-attitudes.

Roulet, T. (2020, December 1). There is another epidemic in the workplace: The domino effect of burn-outs. *Forbes*. www.forbes.com/sites/thomasroulet/2020/12/01/there-is-another-epidemic-in-the-workplacethe-domino-effects-of-burn-outs/?sh=4f44f2e92b1e.

Shaw, G. (2012, July 31). Most adverse events at hospitals still go unreported. The Hospitalist.org. Retrieved from www.the-hospitalist.org/hospitalist/article/125141/most-adverse-events-hospitals-still-go-unreported.

Tariq, R. A., Vashisht, R., Sinha, A., & Scherbak, Y. (2021). *Medication Dispensing Errors and Prevention*. StatPearls (online). Treasure Island, FL: StatPearls Publishing. Retrieved March 5, 2021, from https://pubmed.ncbi.nlm.nih.gov/30085607/.

Tejos, R., Navia, A., Cuadra, A., Fernandez-Diaz, O. F., & Berner, J. E. (2020). Avoiding a second wave of medical errors: The importance of human factors in the context of a pandemic. *Aesthetic Plastic Surgery*, *44*(5), 1926–1928.

US NRC. (2020). Licensing process for operators. www.nrc.gov/reactors/operator-licensing/licensing-process.html.

Veazie, S., Peterson, K., & Bourne, D. (2019). *Evidence Brief: Implementation of High Reliability Organization Principles*. Washington, DC: Department of Veterans Affairs. Retrieved from www.ncbi.nlm.nih.gov/books/NBK542883/.

Zavala, A. M., Day, G. E., Plummer, D., & Bamford-Wade, A. (2018). Decision-making under pressure: Medical errors in uncertain and dynamic environments. *Australian Health Review*, *42*(4), 395–402.

CHAPTER 4

Sources of Medical Error

Yeah, medical errors happen. We do everything we can to avoid them, but they happen. The key is to clean up our messes before they become everyone else's problem as well.

—Internal medicine physician

For me, sometimes when errors occur we really don't have time to consider how or why. That comes later. At that moment, we're just focused on saving the patient.

—Perfusionist

Now that we have discussed the various types of medical errors, we will now more broadly consider the sources of these errors. Why do they occur at all? What actions, contexts, issues, and events make it more likely that a misdiagnosis, a misinterpreted test, an incorrect drug administration, or a wrong-site surgery will occur? We have identified the following general sources as main contributors to error: systems issues, team issues, and individual issues. Clearly, these categories of error source are not mutually exclusive, and in real incidents, the root cause of the failure is often in more than one of these categories. As we have noted, accidents are by far usually the result of a chain of errors rather than a single failure; they have multiple causes rather than some single cause; and the chain of errors could almost always have been interrupted at any of a number of points in the accident scenario. However, it is useful to consider these error sources separately for purposes of analysis, in order to better understand how and why they occur.

Systems Factors

"Systems" refers broadly to the environment in which work takes place, including, among other elements, the physical workplace, tools and equipment, processes and procedures/protocols, and workflows with which healthcare workers operate. We will call systems at this level "local" systems. They represent the most immediate, proximal environment in which healthcare workers perform their duties. Beyond such local workplace systems, though, there are also broader legal, governmental, regulatory, and societal systems that we will call "broader" systems. They are the outermost layers of influence that impact the work of healthcare providers. The most effective local systems are engineered to minimize the likelihood of error consistent with the requirements of the broader systems in which they operate. System-based errors originate when local systems and their superordinate broader systems are not designed for efficient and effective operation, making errors committed by teams or individuals ultimately more likely. Many sources identify system shortcomings on both of the levels we outline here as the primary source of medical error. Systems problems not only have a major impact on team and individual contributing factors; they are also harder for teams or individuals to address directly at the point of healthcare delivery. We will have much more to say on this point later.

Traditionally, when an accident occurs in any setting, the most common first response is to attempt to reengineer the immediate work situation and improve other local system factors to make that particular accident less likely to occur in the future. "Look to the (local) system" is the common first response after an accident. Consider the following typical examples. A factory worker gets a bad cut, and after the investigation, management puts up machine guards and better signage around the equipment in question and establishes new work protocols (standard operating procedures). A pedestrian is struck at an unmarked intersection and local authorities put up crosswalks with flashing lights and warning signs at that intersection. Pilots fail to respond to a three-second auditory emergency alarm in the cockpit, so manufacturers reengineer that alarm to stay on until it is acknowledged and physically silenced by pilots (they might also have been required to do so by new government regulations). Wrong-site surgeries occur in the OR, and the hospital starts requiring patients and/or doctors in consultation to mark the correct site preoperatively with a Sharpie. It is commonplace and absolutely appropriate for investigators to look to systems improvements after an accident as a key to safer performance. There are certainly other contributing causes and prospective solutions, but it is a critical piece of the puzzle to engineer systems to make safe operation easier and errors less likely.

Incident reporting, which perhaps might be more accurately described as underreporting, is an especially critical local-systems issue in healthcare.

While other HROs have built reasonably effective reporting systems to help identify patterns of errors (where, when, and how they occur, who is involved, etc.), healthcare has been comparatively slow to develop accurate and thorough incident reporting processes. Even fatal events are not always captured and coded properly so that they can become a learning experience. Other adverse events, including close calls or near misses, commonly go completely unrecorded. Overall, the healthcare literature indicates that the vast majority of such error-driven events are not accurately and completely captured by existing reporting systems.

Underreporting is inadvertently supported by the legalistic environment in which doctors and other healthcare professionals operate. This broader systems issue will be all too familiar to readers of this book. Fear of litigation and the negative consequences associated with an adverse outcome help support a work culture that keeps errors hidden (Morrison, Cope, & Murray, 2018; Shaw, 2017). In healthcare as well as other HROs, attitudes toward error too often end up framing error as a weakness and/or failure, as well as a source of shame and potential blame and punishment. Fear and other similar negative emotions, as psychologists like John and Joe know, are powerful motivators to avoid doing things, including reporting when things are not quite right (off-normal conditions, unsafe acts), not only after an accident, but even before an accident occurs (e.g., close call/near-miss reporting).

Workload is obviously also a major systems issue. Healthcare providers in every aspect of healthcare work under mounting pressures for productivity. Most industries increasingly expect associates to do more with less, when the reality may be that associates who are experiencing burnout are more likely do less with less, and with more stress. Recall that in earlier chapters we have identified workload as one of the major general contributors to the risk of burnout in any work setting. It is telling that without exception, all of the healthcare professionals we interviewed identified excessive workload (including increasingly rapid pace required, lack of time to double-check, and other indicators of overwork) as a major source of stress in their professional (and then personal) lives.

In some cases, healthcare providers do not have effective protocols, or they fail to follow them if they exist. Paradoxically, *overreliance* on protocols that obviously cannot anticipate every possible consequence can lead to error as well. While protocols are helpful in routinizing work, no protocol can anticipate and apply to every possible situation. The protocol has to be judged to fit the situation, and if it does not, the protocol must be flexibly adapted to fit. Also, while aimed at promoting safe and efficient operation, protocols (e.g., checklists) can lead to a kind of "automation complacency," wherein we may come to rely on the checklist somewhat mindlessly even in an unusual situation. Checklists can be a masterful resource for mitigating errors, especially if they are updated and kept current, but following them without questioning them where they don't fit is also a source of potential error and eventual accident.

Another major broader systems issue in modern healthcare, one that we have touched on earlier as a sore spot for healthcare providers, is the widespread use of electronic health records (EHR). While intended to reduce error, EHR requirements add substantially to physicians' workload and take away from their precious clinical contact time with their patients (Hill, Sears, & Melanson, 2013). As with other industries that have implemented automated systems, while these systems may well result in fewer errors overall, they don't completely eliminate errors and can shift the pattern of the ones that do occur. A keystroke error, for example, is still an error that can have serious consequences in automated systems.

An example from aviation can demonstrate how this automation-based "error shift" takes place. Several decades ago, there began a major engineering movement in aviation to computerize as much of the job of the pilots as possible. The development of the so-called glass cockpit was aimed at reducing pilot error (whether team-based or individual), by having the technology fly the plane. Today, most full-sized commercial aircraft are heavily computerized, and with better engines, better display and control systems, and so on, the glass cockpit has made flying much safer. But errors still occur. A classic and tragic example is Korean Airlines flight 007. In September 1983, a Boeing 747 jumbo jet had unintentionally flown well off-course on its way from Anchorage to Seoul. The crew made a series of uncorrected errors that resulted in incorrectly programming the route and failing to notice that they were far off their intended flight plan and straying into Soviet airspace. Whatever the cause, the crew clearly lacked situational awareness, likely due at least in part to the assumption that the machine was handling it. This was a classic and tragic example of "automation complacency." When the crew failed to respond to attempts by the Soviet pilots to contact them, a missile was launched, KAL 007 was downed, and all souls were lost (Kello, 2017).

Back to the healthcare setting. John has been seeing a specialist off and on for several years. John has commented that he has no idea what color this doctor's eyes are, as the doctor spends most of their few minutes of clinical time during an office visit staring at his laptop, entering notes. Eye contact? Not so much. Not to mention that the growing popularity of telemedicine (even before the pandemic) has further increased the use of technology as opposed to live doctor-patient clinical interactions.

Doctors cannot be replaced with computers. But the assumption that the doctor is infallible and therefore must always be right can lead to a final critical systems issue for us to consider: the status hierarchy in the medical setting. The status hierarchy in the medical setting, as well as in other settings, positions the doctor as the leader with others (e.g., nurses, medical assistants) generally subordinate to the doctor. There are implicit rules (and sanctions) about speaking up to or correcting "the boss." This hierarchy is a systems issue (and also a team issue, as we will see shortly) that in itself can allow error to go unchecked. In his research with the airlines, John has literally heard a first officer say about a captain, "If he made a mistake I would look out the window and hope for the best rather than speak up and identify the error." While that may be an exaggeration (though others in the meeting nodded in agreement), it points to how steep the hierarchy can be in settings like aviation and healthcare.

The bottom line is, even in the best-designed and most fail-safe of systems, errors can and do still occur. And while it is important to continually fine-tune systems for safe operation at the broader and local levels to the extent possible, systems flaws are certainly not the only cause of error and accidents. The effective use of well-designed systems still depends critically on the situational awareness, communication, and coordination of the team of human operators, and the overall fitness for duty of the individuals working within those systems. Let's look at some of the critical team factors as additional potential sources of error.

Teamwork Factors

Regardless of the effectiveness of the systems in place, it is possible for error to occur simply as a result of poor teamwork – even among a group of the most skilled and fit professionals. This may seem paradoxical, as teams are supposed to enhance the effectiveness of the work they perform and to reduce error, just as well-designed systems are. Individual members of the team may be doing well with the information they are given and working within the constraints of their policies and procedures and other systems factors, but failures to communicate updated information as conditions change, failures to watch out for each other, and failures to coordinate actions in a timely manner can result in error regardless. Operating on the basis of assumptions rather than double-checking information can be deadly. It is surprising to many who review accident reports in any industry that so many accidents are primarily the result of team members not being on the same page, or not having a "shared mental model," to use the common expression in the literature on teams. In such cases, it is not only that operators are not working collaboratively and in concert; they may even be working at cross purposes, as was the case in the Three Mile Island nuclear incident. That incident is a textbook example of highly technically trained individual operators lacking that critical shared mental model, with no one calling a time-out to discuss the questions "What do we all know? What's the big picture? Let's pause and think."

John has taken students to a training center with a high-fidelity simulator at a local nuclear power plant to see teamwork in action. John helped establish the training for licensing classes of operators, and among other team skills, emphasized the critical importance of the shared mental model. We must all know what each of us knows. The students are always impressed when, in the course of dealing with an "evolution" (off-normal scenario) in the simulator, an operator raises their hand and calls out, "Update." The whole control room team stops what they were doing individually and comes together to huddle in the middle of the room where team members share information to the point that they literally all now know what each of them knows.

Note that there is a positional leader in the nuclear control room team and a hierarchical management structure in place. In the early days of nuclear operations, the shift supervisor with a senior reactor operator license and management authority mostly told the rest of the team what to do. He (almost always a male) read procedural steps out to the operators, and they performed the actions they were directed to. It was unlikely that an operator would speak out and "challenge" a direction from the boss, even if a possible error was detected. Now admittedly, some supervisors made it easier for operators to speak up, to "have voice," as we now say, but power-sharing and collaborative teamwork were not in the job description. Historically, this local-system hierarchy in the control room was comparable to that in aviation and in healthcare. The boss gives directions and team members follow them.

When John began introducing concepts of teamwork into the control room setting of his local public utility many years ago, he initially observed a mixed reaction. The operators generally loved the idea of being able to speak up, and some of the supervisors accepted some level of power-sharing and real collaboration, but there was concern that the government regulators (i.e., the Nuclear Regulatory Commission) and local management would not take kindly to a "boss" asking his direct reports for input.

As in the airline industry, the leadership role was based on a military model (in the case of the airlines, the captain role was actually based on old maritime law, giving the ship's captain sole legal authority while at sea), and the system expected the supervisor to be in charge and direct the operators, not to ask for their opinions, which would look weak. It took time, but, gradually, the governmental and local systems embraced a shared-leadership model of true teamwork, very different from the classical "command-and-control" role of the supervisor. The results of harnessing the power of the team have been impressive in that industry.

The key to teamwork in any setting is communication. Especially in a highly technical, highly complex HRO work environment such as healthcare, it is easy for the technical professionals to operate in a somewhat isolated fashion, or, to use the common term, "in a silo." The surgeon's role is different from that of the anesthesiologist or the scrub nurse, and these distinctive roles are expected to work in harmony with the other roles for the benefit of the patient. But for that goal of collaborative, mutually supportive teamwork to be reached, there must be clear, relevant, ongoing, and verified communication in order to facilitate coordination of actions. Saying "Update" is a prime example of such communication.

So, what teamwork factors might contribute to error, and why do they occur?

Recognizing the status hierarchy in healthcare teams and other HRO teams, the team leader bears major responsibility for establishing the operating principles of the team at the very outset. The leader must clearly identify expectations (Why are we here? What are we supposed to do? What outcomes are we going to achieve?), role differentiation among team members (Who does what to contribute to the whole?), procedures (What steps we will go through?), and assessment (How did we do against our objectives?). Without this clarification, errors will almost certainly occur. A lack of leader-identified expectations boils down to failures in communication at the outset, along the way, and at the conclusion of an operational procedure.

Not all team leaders are schooled in best-practice techniques of team leadership. They do not fully appreciate the importance of a "team formation" briefing or any other aspect of team leadership. Similar to the way that supervisors in many industries get that leadership role without any specific training in leadership or effective management, many healthcare team leaders are trained in the technical aspects of their role but not in the equally critical teamwork aspects.

Among the eight common root causes of medical errors listed by the Agency for Healthcare Research and Quality, several of the most critical ones are squarely teamwork-based (AHRQ, 2003). For example, the agency report identifies "communication breakdowns" as the most common cause of medical errors. Such breakdowns occur in oral and/or written communication between physician, nurse, healthcare team member, and/or patient. Similarly, the study identifies "inadequate information flow" as a serious contributing factor, arising when necessary information that is needed for accurate medication prescribing is not shared, test results are not adequately shared, or in general when critical information does not follow the patient when they are transferred or discharged. It is fair to say that communication failures are a primary source of teamwork-related errors.

Teamwork breakdowns are prominent among the causes of medical error and, as noted, are considered by at least some sources as the most critical. It is certainly possible for team dysfunction to create error, even when systems factors are effective and supportive of safe work. And we emphasize again, especially in teams where there is a strong positional hierarchy, that it is the role of the team leader to avoid such dysfunction.

Individual Factors

Despite their high level of technical expertise, even the best doctors make mistakes. Even under optimal conditions, we all slip up at times. They may be working within expertly designed systems, and they may have a competent leader and competent teammates who communicate and coordinate well within the team, but individual "person factors" can still cause them to make errors of commission (doing the wrong thing) or errors of omission (failing to do the right thing) at any point in the treatment sequence. The individual-based, person factors can fairly be summed up as "fitness for duty" or lack of same.

To be fit for duty, an individual must have the requisite knowledge and skill to be able to perform their job effectively. They must be well trained and retain the contents of the training as they put that information into practice. Frankly, lack of knowledge is seldom a major problem for physicians and other healthcare providers. Their extensive training, combined with the cognitive abilities required to complete a demanding major and to be accepted into a professional school and complete their training, means that errors are rarely the result of lack of knowledge or technical skill. Now, they may see situations they have never encountered and make a factual error or an error of judgment. But most medical errors are not the result of deficits of knowledge or skill.

In other HROs like aviation and nuclear operations, in addition to extensive initial licensing training, operators are regularly refreshed in the classroom (nuclear) and in simulators (nuclear and aviation). They are also checked in real-time operations at intervals (e.g., a check airman flying with a pilot and copilot), as well as checking their knowledge and skill (e.g., a senior reactor operator assessing individual team members' work). Operators are retrained on critical skills, observed and checked during normal operations, and exposed to emergency, off-normal situations in simulators. The goal of such continual training and checking is to ensure that operators are current in their knowledge and skill and can put that knowledge and skill into action in dealing with challenging situations as well as normal operations. They must individually know what to do and how to do it.

While doctors and other medical experts may not have their training "refreshed," updated, and extended by hours and hours of ongoing class-room and simulator training, regional and national professional conferences expose them to new ideas and current best practices. Additionally, many organizations and hospital systems enable or even require continuing medical education to keep physicians and medical personnel trained up on the latest developments in their practice. So again, lack of knowledge or skill is rarely a root cause of medical error. It can happen, of course, but it is not common. The fitness for duty factor of adequate knowledge and skill is usually positive. Still, as a systems issue, the lack of "continuing education" and training/retraining, work in a simulator, and checking by senior practitioners is a potential gap in healthcare, unlike what is seen in other HROs.

A second critical fitness-for-duty requirement, beyond knowledge and skill, is that the individual be physically and psychologically well. If operators in any field are ill, injured, distracted, or stressed (much less truly burned out), they cannot effectively put their knowledge and skill into practice. They cannot effectively use the system tools they are given or work around inadequate systems support. They cannot individually contribute effectively to, or help harness the power of, the team.

Setting aside physical ailments, consider the psychological effects of burnout. As we have identified throughout this book, our individual risk of making errors is enhanced dramatically under conditions of fatigue, stress, and, of course, the ultimate outcome of prolonged, excessive, unmanaged workplace stress: burnout. Of the many negative effects of the syndrome of burnout, one that is especially problematic and the one that is absolutely central to the purpose of this book is the increased likelihood of error. Stressed-out, burned-out doctors are thereby more prone to make mistakes – not because they lack proper training and understanding of best practices in dealing with a patient problem, nor because their teammates are not communicating, nor because they are working in flawed systems, but because they are individually not fit for duty.

An individual factor that has an interesting history in the safety literature is "accident proneness," that is, the hypothesized propensity for certain personality types to be more at risk for an accident than others. The data are not crystal clear, but some personality factors like aggressiveness, overconfidence, impulsivity, and, in terms of the Five Factor Model of personality, low conscientiousness, high openness, and agreeableness have been suggested as making the individual more likely to be careless than others. Other research has implicated the Type A personality (competitive, impatient, angry-hostile) as the accident-prone type.

Anecdotally, our reviews of archived accident data in industrial settings have found that the same individual may indeed be involved in multiple incidents. For example, John conducted a review of approximately 200 recordable incidents that occurred over a twenty-year period in one industrial company and found that some individuals accounted for as many as four or five of those incidents. Put differently, 150 of those recordables might have occurred with 150 different individuals, but the remaining 50 involved only 12 people, and 5 people accounted for 30 of those 50. Admittedly, time-in-service is a factor. An employee who has worked at the location for twenty years has a greater chance of multiple injuries than an employee who has been there for two years. The long tenure of the twenty-year employee adds an additional risk of complacency, as the senior employee may have done the same task hundreds and hundreds of times before without injury. But even when it is possible to factor out years of service, a few individuals account for more than their share of errors leading to accidents.

During his work as an environmental, health, and safety consultant, John has had the opportunity to attend dozens of accident investigations and reviews in a wide variety of industries. Where relevant, individuals who suffered the accident and/or were primarily responsible for the error that led to the accident are always thoroughly interviewed as part of the accident investigation. In each and every such interview that John has attended, the individual most immediately responsible for the error knew exactly what they did wrong.

Here is a typical Q&A with the employee who suffered a major at-work injury, say, a serious fall while working atop a railcar.

Q: Did you have the proper safety training for working on an elevated platform?
A: Yes, I knew that I was supposed to be harnessed and tied off, and I know the proper procedure for doing that. We get that training in safety meetings a lot.
Q: Did you have the proper PPE?
A: Yes.
Q: Was it in good working order?
A: Yes.
Q: Did you use it?
A: No.
Q: Why not?
A: I was just going to be up there for a minute, and I didn't see the need to add time to the job by going through all that for just a quick up and down. Plus, I have been up on cars hundreds and hundreds of times, and I never fell before. We were behind and I was in a hurry to get caught up.
Q: Did your supervisor or a coworker see you up there without your protective equipment?
A: No, my partner called off sick today, and I was working alone.
Q: What should you have done?
A: Not get in a hurry, go get my harness and use it no matter what, even if I am only up there for ten seconds. I just wasn't thinking. Again, I work up on railcars all the time, and I never had a problem before.

We emphasize again that a doctor experiencing burnout is especially error-prone even if well trained and even when systems and team factors are optimal. No system and no team are perfect, and individual errors can slip through. But in many cases – perhaps most cases – systems and teamwork factors are in fact not always 100 percent optimal, especially in complex situations where events may be off-normal and changing rapidly. More commonly, a medical accident review finds that, let's say, one or more system flaws combined with communication errors and fatigued doctors are the ultimate causes of the adverse event. Note too the critical point that the key to correcting systems flaws and teamwork breakdowns is individual behavior. Alert, mindful individual behavior is that much more difficult to achieve when someone is experiencing burnout.

Turning to Solutions

The healthcare system is in need of solutions that deploy a combination of improved systems (protocols, procedures, technologies, regulations), team factors (communication, coordination, double-checking, watching out for all), and individual factors (fitness for duty, mindfulness, alertness, awareness of how and where error occurs). All of these areas are important. We have emphasized that systems-level shortcomings can negatively impact teamwork and individual performance, and some sources target systems improvements, which impact team and individual performance, as the most critical. Other sources, as we have noted, point to the team as the critical level for managing error and performing safely. We can also make the case that if there is a single one that is most critical, and most closely and directly under the control of the individual healthcare worker, it would be heightened awareness, knowledge, and emotional and physical fitness for duty on the part of every individual on the healthcare team. Working well with existing systems, compensating for systems flaws, and/or correcting systems problems ultimately depends on individual behavior. Similarly, working well within the team or compensating for teamwork errors and correcting them ultimately depends on individual behavior. The key to error management is individual intervention *and* ensuring that the individual is fully fit for duty, working safely, helping the team do so, and making systems improvements to the extent possible. A burned-out physician *is not* fully fit for duty and likely needs individual, team, and system-level intervention to help them return to 100 percent. Thus, the balance of this book turns to and focuses on what we propose as the "solutions" to address such errors. In the next chapters, we emphasize evidence-based individual, team, and system-level solutions that are known to help minimize burnout and the resulting negative consequences including, prominently, errors.

The COVID-19 Effect

Numerous sources have identified the enhanced risks of medical error associated with the pandemic (Ellis, Hay-David, & Brennan, 2020; Hay-David et al., 2020). Many doctors found themselves working in dramatically off-normal conditions and in situations and with equipment with which they are less familiar. As one dramatic and now-common example, operating with full PPE (face shields, respirators) can itself increase the chances of individual error. Quoting from an article from the *British Journal of Oral and Maxillofacial Surgery* (Ellis, Hay-David, & Brennan, 2020):

> Burn out amongst clinicians may become more common in such a demanding environment. It is important that we look out for this in ourselves and our colleagues, recognizing and dealing with this early before it can lead to suboptimal performance. Many clinicians are away from families in order to avoid risk to loved ones. There are also more widespread concerns causing stress and anxiety: COVID-19 testing (patients and healthcare workers);

distrust of governmental decisions; unnecessary "fake" news and scaremongering; concern over inconsistent policies by different trusts in the UK on PPE use (WHO standards versus PHE advice); concern for an overstretched health service that cannot deliver care; and, normal concerns for their own heath and that of their families. Trusts have access to support for healthcare workers suffering from burn out which should be utilised at the earliest opportunity.

All of these factors increase burnout and the risk of medical error. But as noted earlier, there are no data of which we are aware tying the increased likelihood of errors to system factors only or mainly. The error sources interact continually, such that the types of factors identified in the study cited above impact teamwork, and certainly affect the performance of the individual healthcare provider.

Key Takeaways

- Medical errors may be occurring at a lower rate than in the past, as the extent of medical error has become more visible and more widely discussed, and as protocols and techniques to reduce them have been more widely implemented. But given the complexities of diagnosis, treatment, and follow-up, and the tens of thousands of daily interactions between patient and doctor, nurse, and pharmacist, errors still occur on a large scale.
- Primary sources of error are systems (both local workplace policies and procedures as well as broader societal and governmental requirements and technological advancements), teamwork, and individual factors.
- A case can be made for each of these error sources being most critical, but the reality is that they all interact. Poor systems factors make it harder for teams to work effectively and make it more likely that the individual will make mistakes. Poor teamwork puts additional stress on individuals. Fatigued, burned-out individuals are likely to be less effective team members and may misuse or otherwise violate existing systems designed for safe and effective operation.

REFERENCES

AHRQ. (2003). AHRQ's patient safety initiative: building foundations, reducing risk. Retrieved March 8, 2021, from https://archive.ahrq.gov/research/findings/final-reports/pscongrpt/psini2.html.

Ellis, R., Hay-David, A. G. C., & Brennan, P. A. (2020). Operating during the COVID-19 pandemic: How to reduce medical error. *British Journal of Oral*

and Maxillofacial Surgery, 58(5), 577–580. doi: https://doi.org/10.1016/j
.bjoms.2020.04.002.
Hay-David, A. G. C., Herron, J. B. T., Gilling, P., Miller, A., & Brennan, P. A.
(2020). Reducing medical error during a pandemic. *British Journal of Oral and
Maxillofacial Surgery, 58*(5), 581–584. doi: 10.1016/j.bjoms.2020.04.003.
Hill, R. G., Jr., Sears, L. M., & Melanson, S. W. (2013). 4000 clicks:
A productivity analysis of electronic medical records in a community hospi-
tal ED. *The American Journal of Emergency Medicine, 31*(11), 1591–1594.
Kello, J. E. (2017). The machine will handle it … right? Automation doesn't
replace the need for vigilance. *Industrial Safety & Hygiene News,* 51(4), 16.
Morrison, M., Cope, V., & Murray, M. (2018). The underreporting of medica-
tion errors: A retrospective and comparative root cause analysis in an acute
mental health unit over a 3-year period. *International Journal of Mental
Health Nursing, 27*(6), 1719–1728. doi:10.1111/inm.12475.
Shaw, G. (2017). Most adverse events at hospitals still go unreported. The
Hospitalist.org. Retrieved from www.the-hospitalist.org/hospitalist/article/
125141/most-adverse-events-hospitals-still-go-unreported.

CHAPTER 5

How-To Strategies for Addressing the Crisis
Solution #1: Understand Your Personality

> I have to get my mind off of work. At home, "talk about work for 15 minutes, then no more." Exercise when I can . . . talk with old friends from pharmacy school. . . .
>
> —Pharmacist

> At the micro-personal level, take time off, reduce your load, spend time with the family (social support), exercise . . . get clear on "what's important to me" . . . change your approach, or get another job.
>
> —Medical school professor

As we have shown throughout this book so far, burnout among physicians and other healthcare providers is a growing crisis not only for practitioners at all levels but potentially for their patients as well. In this and the forthcoming chapters, we turn our attention to strategies to reduce the likelihood of burnout and therefore the likelihood of medical error. Effective strategies exist at the level of individuals, teams, and systems, and of course none of these operates in isolation – indeed, these strategies continually interact. We will discuss this interactive perspective later. For now, to better understand each of these lines or levels of attack on the burnout crisis, we will discuss them separately.

Specifically, the first four solutions that we propose (Chapters 5–8) will relate to individual-level strategies, while the following three chapters (Chapters 9–11) focus on team-level solutions and strategies. The next four chapters (Chapters 12–15) focus on organization, management, and other "local" system-level solutions, as well as "broader" system-level solutions including national healthcare policies and regulations. The goal is to provide a multilevel framework of solutions (i.e., individual, team, system) that can assist physicians and healthcare workers across the board in managing their stress. We must emphasize again that no single solution or solution at a single level of attack has the power to completely resolve or even significantly mitigate the burnout issue. Deploying multiple solutions will be necessary.

To begin, let's look first at individual-level solutions, which are those solutions most directly under the control of the individual. Physicians and other healthcare providers can take these actions right now without supervisor permission, enhanced teamwork, organizational policy changes, or legislative interventions. Our interviewees identified these practices first and foremost when we asked, "What can be done now to reduce the risk of burnout or the level of burnout for you?" Further, these solutions are most directly tied to the psychological experience of burnout, as we have defined it. In a sense they are the first best line of defense against burnout.

The primary predictor of the burnout syndrome, by definition, is prolonged, excessive, work-related stress that is not successfully managed. Therefore, one major key to buffering the individual against the risk of burnout is stress management by the individual. Fortunately, there is an extensive scientific and practical literature on stress and stress management that stretches back over the past hundred years (at least). Over the next few chapters that focus on individual-level strategies and solutions for mitigating burnout, we will (1) briefly overview critical elements of the literature on personality that pertain to burnout risk and (2) emphasize the individually controlled health-promoting activities that can help mitigate stress and reduce or eliminate burnout.

Understand Your Personality

"Know thyself." This adage encompasses the first major solution at the individual level. Some personality traits predispose one to burnout, while other traits are associated with reduced risk. Before we explore the traits in question, let's first be clear on what we mean by "personality." In behavioral science, personality refers to the structures, propensities, and traits of a person that explain their characteristic patterns of emotion, behavior, and thought (Funder, 2001). More specifically, personality is the distinctive patterns of thought and behavior that remain relatively consistent for an individual across situations and over time. This durable pattern of behavior and thinking influences how the individual is perceived by others and, to a considerable extent, also impacts how they adjust to the demands of their work and to their social environments. Personality is reflected in such familiar everyday statements as: "I'm a detail person," "I'm a people person," "My friend is just so thoughtful," "You are a dependable, hard worker," "They have a great sense of humor." People frequently use these kinds of statements to describe someone, essentially, describing their perceptions of a person's consistent and distinctive traits across situations and over time, that is, their personality.

Personality traits help to determine whether one can interact with another person effectively. That other person has their personality characteristics as well, of course, and they may be quite different. Personality conflicts arise when two people have fundamentally different and incompatible personality traits, and their behaviors are at odds. This is what is colloquially known as a "personality clash." Joe and John both commiserate about certain professional collaborators with whom they just could not work effectively, not because the person was necessarily a bad person, but because their style of working and interacting was so different from ours.

Next, let's investigate what personality theorists and researchers have had to say about the basic dimensions and fundamental traits of personality. It is an understatement to say that psychologists have taken a multitude of approaches to understanding the fundamental dimensions of personality over many years. The most studied and the widely cited personality framework, as well as the one with the most contemporary scientific empirical support, is the Five Factor Model (FFM), also known as the "Big Five" personality model. The five fundamental personality factors identified in this predominant contemporary model are conscientiousness, agreeableness, neuroticism, openness (to experience), and extraversion (Barrick & Mount, 1991). The model is so widely cited that many people have heard of the Big Five personality dimensions, be it through formal education (e.g., in introductory psychology courses), leadership workshops, individual leadership coaching, or just conversations with others (like Joe and John) about personality. Each of the Big Five factors has the potential to greatly impact one's susceptibility to, and experience with, burnout. That's the critical point on which we want to elaborate. Here we go.

"Conscientiousness" refers to the tendency to display self-discipline, to act dutifully, and to strive for achievement (DeYoung, Quilty, & Peterson, 2007). The job market particularly seeks applicants with this personality trait, with organizations paying good money for selection measures to identify applicants who are high in conscientiousness. Those who are high in conscientiousness tend to be organized and show a strong preference for control over their environment. We all know folks who are highly conscientious, and we may even describe some of them as uptight and perfectionistic; for example, when we move a book on their shelf they promptly fix it before carrying on the conversation (true story). Conscientiousness in that extreme form, however, can prove problematic for stress and subsequent burnout.

"Agreeableness" reflects concern for social harmony (Graziano, Jensen-Campbell, & Hair, 1996). A person high in agreeableness is typically warm, kind, cooperative, sympathetic, helpful, and courteous. They see their desire to prioritize supportive communication and to obtain acceptance in interpersonal relationships as an important expression of their personality (Barrick & Mount, 1991). These people tend to try to get along more than get ahead, and may occasionally be taken advantage of for that reason. Someone who is high in agreeableness may experience stress and burnout when they are asked to do more and more tasks without additional resources, time, or money to accomplish those tasks, and they agree to do so. They do not want to disagree or create conflict, as that is inconsistent with their high-agreeableness personality, and so they end up adding more to their plate, potentially to a breaking point. Given the overwhelming pace of work in healthcare, highly agreeable physicians may be at a higher risk of burnout. We must emphasize, though, that the data on agreeableness are mixed, with some studies suggesting that high scores in agreeableness can in fact be a stress buffer.

"Neuroticism" refers to the tendency of an individual to experience and express negative emotions, particularly anger, anxiety, and depression (Barrick & Mount, 1991). In much contemporary research with the Five Factor Model, neuroticism is relabeled as "need for structure" or "need for stability," indicating that high scores in neuroticism on a Big Five test do not automatically indicate a diagnosable form of psychopathology – a neurosis – using the older and familiar terminology. Rather, these scores indicate that the individual is prone to experiencing and expressing negative emotion and may undergo a stronger stress reaction than others in a similar situation. For our discussion of personality traits, we will use the traditional term "neurotic," but only in a general, nonclinical sense. In those terms, people who are highly neurotic in terms of the Five Factor model are nervous, moody, emotional, often jealous, and insecure. From a job perspective, organizations tend to prefer employees who are lower on neuroticism, as they tend to be calmer, steady, and more secure (Barrick & Mount, 2000). However, some research suggests that moderate levels of neuroticism may be associated with high achievement orientation, as anxiety may motivate an individual to work harder, longer, and more consistently. This is particularly the case among graduate students, including medical students (Meyer & Winer, 1993). And yet, at the same time, as the definition makes clear, a high level of neuroticism is more strongly associated with stress-proneness and risk of burnout than any of the other personality characteristics in the Big Five. And again, while high scores in neuroticism are not in and of themselves indicative of psychopathology, high scores in neuroticism do put individuals in a higher risk category for a variety of forms of psychological disorder, from the mild to moderate anxiety and depressive disorders to more severe forms as well.

"Openness to experience" refers to the propensity to appreciate art and adventure, to have unusual ideas, vivid imagination, high levels of curiosity, and a desire for a variety of experiences (Barrick & Mount, 2000). Individuals with more openness to experience are typically more intellectually curious, open to emotion (not just logic), sensitive to beauty, and willing to try new things. They tend to be more creative and more aware of their feelings. People who are more open to experiences tend to prefer jobs and environments that are more fluid and dynamic, with rapid changes in demands (Cellar, Miller, Doverspike, & Klawsky, 1996). They prefer situations where new things happen regularly.

In many ways, high scores in openness may have the potential to buffer against burnout, a notion generally supported by the evidence. Specifically, research has indicated repeatedly that those who are more open are also more tolerant for ambiguity (Furnham & Marks, 2013). They tend not to be as upset, disrupted, or even feel anxious when things go differently than expected or when they are unable to explain a situation. This strong positive relationship between openness to experience and tolerance for ambiguity may buffer burnout when the source is something akin to ambiguity, such as unclear expectations or uncertainty in a patient's diagnosis.

"Extraversion" refers to a trait of individuals who are more talkative, sociable, assertive, bold, passionate, with a tendency to want to dominate situations (Judge, Bono, Ilies, & Gerhardt, 2002). In contrast, introverts (at the low end of the extraversion scale) tend to be more analytical, quiet, shy, and reserved. As a side point, introverts are not unsociable, though the myth of them being unsociable is still present in the popular literature. They are mainly slower to "warm up" and get comfortable in social situations, and not as quick to just dive in, as extraverts are. Extraverted individuals tend to prioritize status and attention, both within their groups and outside their inner circle. This attention-seeking behavior is generally adaptive, but can present some challenges in more egalitarian systems and situations, such as the all-important team setting, where sharing the spotlight is prized over individual achievement. Extraverted individuals tend to be more energetic with an emphasis on quick problem solving, and show a propensity to be optimistic and to experience positive emotions much more than negative. As such, extraversion may be a personality characteristic likely to buffer against stress and burnout for individuals.

Personality and Burnout among Physicians

With these general definitions in mind, we turn our attention to some of the findings relating personality and burnout specifically among physicians and other medical professionals. In an international sample of physicians, Brown and colleagues (2019) consistently found that neuroticism was negatively related to personal accomplishment and positively related to both emotional exhaustion and depersonalization among doctors. Highly neurotic individuals are much more likely to experience all three dimensions of burnout and will need to double-down on their efforts in other areas to mitigate the onset of burnout. Brown and colleagues (2019) also found that agreeableness and conscientiousness were positively related to personal accomplishment and negatively related to both emotional exhaustion and depersonalization. In other words, these two personality characteristics may buffer against the onset and experience of burnout among physicians, while, again, neuroticism may exacerbate burnout.

Although the data in the Brown et al. (2019) study did not show it, based on other data we anticipate that moderate to high levels of extraversion and openness to experience may also help with managing burnout. In both cases contextual factors may be especially important. That is, given their social orientation, extraverts may be more likely to reach out for social support (an especially critical stress buffer). Given their relative comfort with ambiguity, individuals with moderate to high levels of openness may be better positioned to handle that particular job-related stressor.

Furthermore, the pattern of relationships for neuroticism found in the Brown et al. (2019) study was confirmed in studies with medical residents in all specialties (Prins et al., 2019), nurses (Divinakumar et al., 2019), and anesthesiologists (Van der Wal et al., 2016). In general, across the full set of Big Five personality factors, some have the potential to buffer against burnout (e.g., agreeableness and conscientiousness, and especially in certain contexts extraversion and openness), while one in particular, namely, neuroticism, is consistently shown to be problematic.

If you have never taken one of the Big Five assessments, you may still have a good sense of your strongest traits from the description we have provided. You will likely have recognized at least parts of yourself in our thumbnail sketch of the defining characteristics of each of the factors. If you have interest in seeing your personality profile in more detail, there are numerous "short forms" of personality assessments anchored to the Five Factor Model available online at no cost. The following is a link to a popular site that offers an assessment along with some interpretation (Truity, 2021): www.truity.com/test/big-five-personality-test.

The Truity website offers a free and user-friendly version of the Big Five personality test that you can take within minutes. As an overview for those who may be interested, the test comprises a series of potentially self-descriptive statements that the test-taker scores as accurate (in describing the self), neutral, or inaccurate, on a five-point scale, followed by a series of potentially self- descriptive adjectives that the test taker self-assesses on the same scale. Once the test is completed, it is immediately automatically scored, each factor of the Big Five is rated on a percentile scale, and a brief explanation of each factor is given.

Work-Around Strategies

So, let's say you identify that you are very low in conscientiousness or very high in neuroticism. Let's say further that those traits are not beneficial to you in your professional and personal roles. Are those less-than-effective tendencies a "sentence" for burnout, leaving you with nothing you can do? The short answer is "No." The longer answer is "No, no, not at all."

An apt analogy compares personality preferences (and measured traits are really just preferences) to handedness. Most of us are firmly right-handed. Writing, throwing a ball, holding a fork, brushing our teeth, and so on are done with the right hand. That is our clear preference. But what if we were unable to use the right hand to carry out those activities, let's say, due to an injury? We use the left hand. It is a bit awkward and takes practice, but we can do it. In fact, if we do it long enough it becomes less uncomfortable. That simple analogy helps us understand that a personality trait is a preference, not a limitation. We can learn what are called "work-around" strategies. Say I am introverted, and I realize that my professional and personal life require that I engage with people, attend social functions, take leadership roles at times, speak up, go first – then, what do I do? I look at what extraverted people do naturally and adopt some of that (left-handed) behavior. Speaking up in group meetings is behavior I can learn, even if it is not the effortless, natural, first impulse for me. I can think it through in advance and plan and prepare to speak up. The same is true for all our personality traits. They are preferences that represent our comfort zones, not limitations. This is a critical point.

As we have noted, there is good research to support the idea that medical practitioners who are low in neuroticism and high in conscientiousness and extraversion (and possibly agreeableness) are naturally more prone to better stress management and a lower risk of burnout. But those who are the opposite in terms of personality factors are not automatically destined to suffer burnout. However, it is to their advantage to identify the specific work-arounds that demonstrate lower neuroticism and higher conscientiousness and extraversion characteristics. Just as the introvert can learn to "put on some of the behavior of the extravert" when it helps them be more effective, so can any of the natural tendencies be offset by learned work-around behavior.

Specifically, and critically, high-neuroticism individuals can recognize that giving in to emotional meltdowns is toxic to themselves and those around them. Lower-neuroticism individuals naturally keep the emotional reaction and expression to a minimum. We will touch on the concept of "constructive self-talk" later in this chapter. For now, just note than it is a common and effective stress-management strategy that is naturally implemented by low-neuroticism individuals. When faced with a challenge, they are naturally prone to say things to themselves (usually not out loud) such as, "You can handle this. It's no big deal, you've seen this before. You know what to do." Such strategies allow them to remain calm and logical. In effect they coach themselves in constructive ways. The good news for high-neuroticism individuals is that the research shows clearly that such self-talk strategies can be taught to and used by anyone, even if it does not come naturally. Constructive self-talk is an especially valuable work-around strategy for high-neuroticism individuals.

Low-conscientiousness individuals can recognize that high-conscientiousness behavior is nearly universally rewarded. Their work-arounds can include setting deadlines for themselves, keeping and updating to-do lists, and in general making certain that they hold themselves fully accountable and honor their commitments. Low-agreeableness individuals can recognize that not every issue has to be debated, and they don't lose anything by going along to get along when the issue at hand is not critical.

There is one final point on the Five Factor Model that is suggested in some of our previous discussion. We do not wish to give the impression that the strongest version of each trait is automatically best. Yes, high-conscientiousness individuals, with their dutifulness and strong achievement striving, are generally effective in their roles at work. But "too much" conscientiousness can result in an inflexible rule-follower or a perfectionist for whom good enough is never good enough. By the same token, "too much" agreeableness can result in individuals being walked on like a doormat and experiencing added stress. Extreme low-neuroticism individuals can come across as unfeeling and uncaring to others. All logic and no feeling can come across like "Mr. Spock" in *Star Trek*. The data suggest strongly that extremely high or extremely low traits are not as effective as "relatively high or relatively low," with versatility in terms of each trait.

Other Personality Characteristics That May Reduce or Enhance Burnout: Beyond the Big Five

While the Big Five has become the most prominent contemporary framework for understanding personality, it is not the only way that personality variables have been identified and studied in the past. Here we overview several of the personality traits that have been identified in the past as relating to stress proneness or stress resistance. As one example, "hardiness" is a variable identified for many decades in stress research as a personality characteristic that enables individuals to manage stress more effectively and to bounce back quickly from stressors, even major ones. Hardiness is very similar to the more contemporary concept of "resilience," which shows up by that name in much contemporary stress research, or, in everyday terms, mental toughness. While not necessarily identical, hardiness does correlate with relatively low neuroticism.

Although hardiness and resilience are personality traits, it is important to recognize there are skills associated with these traits that can be learned and applied by any individual. Just as an introvert can "act" extraverted when they need to, a person can learn the skills associated with resilience and behave accordingly. Because of this, some organizations have started offering resilience training for their employees to assist them in staving off burnout. For example, Martin and colleagues (2019) developed a resilience education and training program based on positive psychological frameworks and deployed the training among healthcare systems in the southeastern United States, with meaningful results. Specifically, they saw a precipitous increase in resilience after the training, and burnout measures also trended lower.

Other identified factors based on older personality research and classifications of traits include self-efficacy, an optimistic explanatory style, an internal locus of control, and a tendency toward constructive self-talk during stressful situations. Self-efficacy is a heavily researched personality characteristic that relates to the individual's belief that they can competently handle a given situation, essentially, that they are effective. Note that reduced self-efficacy is one of the three defining facets of the burnout syndrome. The relationship between self-efficacy and any of the five factors is not obvious, but in general, individuals who are confident in their ability to handle things might be expected to be lower in neuroticism and possibly higher in conscientiousness. An optimistic explanatory style refers to one's tendency to have a positive outlook, expect the best, and frame stressors in less threatening ways. Research shows it is also characteristic of individuals who score high on the extravert scale. We would expect that this characteristic would also overlap with low neuroticism. Internal locus of control (touched on briefly in Chapter 1) is characteristic of individuals who believe that they themselves influence the things that happen to them. They are in control of their lives, not at the mercy of chance events. Connections with the Five Factor Model are not completely clear, though we might comfortably speculate that there might be a relationship between internal locus of control and relatively high conscientiousness scores.

Individuals who possess these personality traits of self-efficacy, optimistic explanatory style, internal locus of control, and a tendency toward constructive self-talk tend not to automatically frame stressors as threats. They do not experience the same intensity of the stress reaction as others do. Individuals with those traits are, to some extent, buffered by the virtue of their positive outlook, natural resilience, belief that they control their fate, and tendency to "coach" themselves through challenges with constructive self-talk. This is good news if one is "wired" that way, but should those of us without these traits resign ourselves to experiencing high levels of stress and high risk for burnout?

The further good news is that while these personality traits are largely innate, "natural" tendencies, these characteristics are all learnable to a significant degree for the rest of us. The concept of work-around strategies, introduced earlier in the context of the Five Factor Model, applies to all personality traits, in whatever way they are conceptualized. Many forms of therapy aimed at reducing anxiety and/or depression focus on so-called cognitive reframing, that is, helping affected individuals think differently about the challenges they face (indeed, which we all face). These are work-around strategies. We also briefly referenced the concept of constructive self-talk above. Let us examine the concept in a bit more detail by illustrating one example of constructive versus negative/dysfunctional self-talk. Initial studies in this area showed a significant correlation between how leaders assessed their direct reports' effectiveness and those direct reports' tendency toward constructive self-talk. More recent work has suggested that constructive self-talk is not just dispositional, hardwired, and immutable, but is to a significant extent teachable and learnable, that is, a work-around. By simply practicing a positive internal monologue during times of stress (e.g., "You've got this! You know you can handle it" or "This is time-limited. You've seen it before") instead of a dysfunctional internal monologue (e.g., "Oh no . . . I don't think I can handle it"), individuals can increase their positivity and reduce their stress reaction substantially.

The Type A Conundrum

Another well-known personality syndrome deserves special attention: the "Type A" personality. Physicians are as likely as anyone else to be optimistic and resilient. They are likely to be confident in their knowledge, skill, and ability to handle anything. They are also likely to show characteristics of the stress-prone Type A personality. This much-researched syndrome was first identified in cardiac patients who had survived a heart attack (Friedman & Rosenman, 1959). Doctors noticed that many of those patients had some personality variables in common that added up to heightened risk for cardiovascular disease. Three contributing facets of the Type A syndrome were then identified as follows: competitiveness, time-urgency, and anger/hostility. Type A patients were prone to strive hard for success, competing both against others and their past performance. To them, everything is a competition that they are driven to win and hate to lose. In addition, these individuals try to do as much as possible in as little time as possible. They stack or nest tasks (so-called multiphasia). They might eat lunch in the car while listening to a self-help tape, all while driving (quickly) to a business meeting. They hate to waste time and they hate to have others waste their time. Finally, and critically, there is the identified "anger-hostility" facet to the Type A personality. If they are, say, thwarted in their attempt to reach a goal, if they lose a "game," or if they get stuck in traffic, they are likely to blow up.

Most research suggests that the actual "cardiac risk factor" for Type As rests on the anger-hostility axis and that competitiveness and time urgency in themselves (typical of high-conscientiousness individuals) do not automatically put one at higher risk for stress-related illness or burnout. But those two more benign facets are predictors of the third, toxic facet. Again, physicians are very likely to have Type A personalities. When they are under pressure, they are prone to just try harder, do more, and do it faster. Type As are also prone to go it alone, bypassing opportunities for that all-critical social support.

If you seem some of yourself in this brief description of Type A, recognize that your drive to do it all, your "workaholism" puts you at higher risk of burnout. It is critically important that you manage the anger that can come with anything that blocks your progress toward your goals.

If anger is in the mix for you, anger management training may be especially important for you.

Summing Up

The most effective strategy for stress management is to implement a combination of strategies. In this chapter, we introduced individual strategies focused on heightened self-awareness. We overviewed personality traits that might make one more or less stress-prone, with an initial focus on the Five Factor Model, which is the most prominent and most thoroughly researched contemporary personality framework. We also identified additional, older approaches to personality that have relevance to stress-proneness and stress-resistance. We identified the importance of developing personality trait "work-around" strategies as needed to minimize stress and the likelihood of burnout. For healthcare providers, the challenge (to borrow a well-known phrase) is to "just do it" and to accept that there are limits to what a doctor or other provider can handle without intentionally applying individual strategies.

The COVID-19 Effect

As the role and responsibility of physicians and other healthcare providers has become ever more stressful in recent decades, the personality-based solutions identified here have long been important. As the pressures of the role have grown, it has become increasingly important that healthcare professionals recognize the stresses they are dealing with and practice the kinds of individual stress-management strategies including the work-around strategies recommended here. All this was true and widely acknowledged before March 2020. But the pandemic dramatically increased the stress level of everyone in the delivery of healthcare. Mitigation strategies have become more important than ever, starting with increased self-awareness and knowledge of our personality-based tendencies. The increased pace and pressure attendant to the pandemic makes it harder than ever to "keep your head down and just get through it."

Key Takeaways

- Different personality traits are associated with reduced or elevated stress reaction. For example, individuals with personality dimensions such as moderately strong extraversion, hardiness, and generalized self-efficacy handle stressful situations better.

• Those who have personalities that predispose them to burnout can use work-around strategies to avoid the deleterious effects.

• Type A personalities are more likely to experience stress and burnout, but they too can benefit more from practicing one or more of the tried and true individual stress-management strategies.

REFERENCES

Barrick, M. R., & Mount, M. K. (1991). The Big Five personality dimensions and job performance: A meta-analysis. *Personnel Psychology, 44*(1), 1–26.

(2000). Select on conscientiousness and emotional stability. In *Handbook of Principles of Organizational Behavior*, ed. M. Hauser and R. J. House (vol. 15, p. 28). Malden, MA: Blackwell.

Brown, P. A., Slater, M., & Lofters, A. (2019). Personality and burnout among primary care physicians: An international study. *Psychology Research and Behavior Management, 12*, 169.

Cellar, D. F., Miller, M. L., Doverspike, D. D., & Klawsky, J. D. (1996). Comparison of factor structures and criterion-related validity coefficients for two measures of personality based on the five factor model. *Journal of Applied Psychology, 81*(6), 694.

DeYoung, C. G., Quilty, L. C., & Peterson, J. B. (2007). Between facets and domains: 10 aspects of the Big Five. *Journal of Personality and Social Psychology, 93*(5), 880.

Divinakumar, K. J., Bhat, P. S., Prakash, J., & Srivastava, K. (2019). Personality traits and its correlation to burnout in female nurses. *Industrial Psychiatry Journal, 28*(1), 24.

Friedman, M., & Rosenman, R. H. (1959). Association of specific overt behavior pattern with blood and cardiovascular findings: Blood cholesterol level, blood clotting time, incidence of arcus senilis, and clinical coronary artery disease. *Journal of the American Medical Association, 169*(12), 1286–1296.

Funder, D. C. (2001). Accuracy in personality judgment: Research and theory concerning an obvious question. In *Personality Psychology in the Workplace*, ed. B. W. Roberts & R. Hogan (pp. 121–140). American Psychological Association.

Furnham, A., & Marks, J. (2013). Tolerance of ambiguity: A review of the recent literature. *Psychology, 4*(9), 717–728.

Graziano, W. G., Jensen-Campbell, L. A., & Hair, E. C. (1996). Perceiving interpersonal conflict and reacting to it: The case for agreeableness. *Journal of Personality and Social Psychology, 70*(4), 820.

Judge, T. A., Bono, J. E., Ilies, R., & Gerhardt, M. W. (2002). Personality and leadership: A qualitative and quantitative review. *Journal of Applied Psychology, 87*(4), 765.

Martin, S., Fiske, B., & Lane, S. (2019). Resilience training for health care professionals. *Journal of Obstetric, Gynecologic & Neonatal Nursing, 48*(3), S94.

Meyer, B. W., & Winer, J. L. (1993). The career decision scale and neuroticism. *Journal of Career Assessment, 1*(2), 171–180.

Prins, D. J., van Vendeloo, S. N., Brand, P. L., van der Velpen, I., de Jong, K., van den Heijkant, F., . . . & Prins, J. T. (2019). The relationship between burnout, personality traits, and medical specialty. A national study among Dutch residents. *Medical Teacher, 41*(5), 584–590.

Truity. (2021, March 2). The Big Five personality test. Retrieved March 9, 2021, from www.truity.com/test/big-five-personality-test.

van der Wal, R. A., Bucx, M. J., Hendriks, J. C., Scheffer, G. J., & Prins, J. B. (2016). Psychological distress, burnout and personality traits in Dutch anaesthesiologists: A survey. *European Journal of Anaesthesiology (EJA), 33* (3), 179–186.

CHAPTER 6

Solution #2: Engage in Self-Care

Probably the worst thing about the long hours is defaulting to whatever the vending machine has in it for my lunch.

—Medical resident

The second solution that we propose at the individual level, and one that a physician or other healthcare worker can do right now, is to engage actively in self-care. Many have attempted to define self-care over the years, with the most prominent definitions coming from the World Health Organization. They define self-care as "what people do for themselves to establish and maintain health, and to prevent and deal with illness. It is a broad concept encompassing hygiene (general and personal), nutrition (type and quality of food eaten), lifestyle (sporting activities, leisure, etc.), environmental factors (living conditions, social habits, etc.), socio-economic factors (income level, cultural beliefs, etc.), and self-medication" (World Health Organization, 1998). More simply stated, self-care is the practice of taking action to improve and preserve one's health and well-being. As we have described the challenges faced by physicians and healthcare workers in terms of working conditions and unique situational factors (prominently, the ongoing global pandemic), it probably comes as no surprise we would encourage them to "take care of yourself, ya hear?!" We note too that such advice is commonly dispensed by physicians and healthcare workers to patients who are under stress, a point we will amplify greatly in an upcoming chapter.

Working from the WHO definition, a variety of lists of the key categories, domains, and pillars of self-care have been developed by researchers (e.g., Selbst & Zultanky, 2020). We provide here an integration of the key elements of these different lists and propose what we will call the "ten pillars" of self-care. We then discuss some additional domains of self-care that may require a bit more attention and clarification.

The Ten Pillars of Self-Care

The International Self-Care Foundation, a charity based in the United Kingdom, works with a variety of stakeholders in health in an effort to provide support to countries, communities, and individuals as they adopt evidence-based self-care practices (ISF, 2020). In their efforts, they identified seven pillars of self-care that encompass physical, emotional, social, and workplace self-care strategies. We provide a summary of these seven pillars here and integrate content from other lists that we discovered in our search for best practices in self-care plans. The result is a list of ten pillars of self-care that we identify as important prescriptions both for overall well-being in general and for reduced stress and risk of burnout in particular (see Table 6.1).

Health literacy: Health literacy refers to the capacity of individuals to obtain access to and understand basic health information. This pillar is superordinate to the others, which is why we address it first. After all, without the relevant information, how could people engage in any of the further self-care strategies provided here and elsewhere? Granted, for the primary audience reading this book, namely, physicians and other health-care workers, we assume you have both access to and understanding of basic health information in general, and particularly as it pertains to stress and burnout. In addition to access and understanding, however, individuals must then actively engage in the processes, procedures, and practices recommended by the health information. The compliance with those principles can mitigate a host of physical as well as emotional problems in general, and we know that physicians are not always the best at following their own advice. John and Joe have been told by doctors and nurses on more than a few occasions that "doctors and nurses make the worst patients." John's wife is a retired nurse. She is one of the resources for the above quote.

Mental well-being: The second pillar of self-care is mental well-being. This pillar comprises psychological health checks, obviously including screening for psychological disorders when deemed appropriate or necessary by a physician, but also including periodic self-assessment. Too often we forget about the psychological aspects of self-care, even when our preclinical/normal-range levels of a potential disorder start to become a bit more clinical. For example, Joe will admit that he has a few preclinical level indicators of obsessive compulsive disorder. Most of the time these traits are adaptive, for example, resulting in increased attention to detail when writing manuscripts or a book for publication. Some measure of

Table 6.1. *The ten pillars of self-care*

	Definition	Example
1. Health literacy	Obtain access to and understand basic health information	Going to a physician and internalizing the care recommendations they make
2. Mental well-being	Cultivate the ability to cope with emotions and stress; encompasses emotional, psychological and social health	Psychological health checks
3. Physical activity	Practice moderate-intensity exercise	Walking, cycling, playing a sport
4. Healthy eating	Have a nutritious, balanced diet, appropriate level of calorie intake	Consuming fruits and vegetables, limiting intake of desserts and refined carbohydrates
5. Risk avoidance or mitigation	Find ways to eliminate risky behavior	Quitting tobacco use, limiting/eliminating alcohol consumption, staying up to date on vaccinations
6. Good hygiene	Maintain physical well-being and appearance through everyday tasks	Hand washing, brushing teeth, washing food before eating
7. Rational and responsible use of products, services, diagnostics, and medicines	Follow recommendations for products, services, diagnostics, and medicines	Avoiding inappropriate usage of prescription medicine, limiting dosages or usage of products to only what is necessary
8. Social self-care	Take actions to increase one's ability to manage stress through building positive social relationships and support	Taking a lunch break to meet a friend, going on a date with your partner, spending time with family
9. Emotional self-care	Take actions that acknowledge the feelings one has related to both positive and negative experiences	Keeping a reflective journal, tracking moods
10. Workplace self-care	Recognize and utilize provisions available at your job to aid in overall wellness	Taking advantage of break room amenities (e.g., coffee), employee assistance programs, lunch and learn sessions

perfectionism can be a good thing indeed! Most of us would prefer to be in the hands of an airline pilot or a surgeon who strives for perfection in their work. We hope that the operators of nuclear power plants have some measure of perfectionism as well! However, such traits can, when carried to extremes (as when under stress), impact life satisfaction. Joe has to be reminded of that from time to time by his social support group (Thank you Joy!). John has no comment here . . .

It is healthy to remember that there is a continuum from low-level, everyday anxiety or mood changes to the extreme forms that are diagnosable as syndromes of psychological disorder. We all know what it's like to have the mild forms. If we are stuck in a tight enough space with a large enough crowd, we can all experience low-grade claustrophobia. But when the "symptoms" start to intensify without any environmental reason, that's the time for a psychological health checkup.

Physical activity: As the third pillar, physical activity refers to practicing moderate-intensity physical activity. This can include walking, cycling, or engaging in a participative sport of some kind. In other words, consistent with a host of research on exercise and well-being (e.g., Klaperski et al., 2019), people need to engage in the self-care strategy of getting up and moving a bit more, rather than the "Netflix and chill" routine (common during the stay-at-home orders of the pandemic) .

Healthy eating: Consistent with the other physical self-care pillars identified here, healthy eating as a pillar of self-care refers to essentially having a nutritious balanced diet, including an appropriate level of caloric intake relative to daily activity levels. In other words, going on yo-yo dieting programs to lose twenty pounds here or there is likely to *not* support self-care strategies when dealing with high levels of stress or burnout. The key is balance, a homeostasis-generating diet (i.e., slowly losing or gaining weight to the desirable spot and stabilizing) that does not create the physical issues and emotional challenges of the ups and downs of general dieting. Consistent healthy eating, and moderation in the intake of unhealthy food and drink, is the key.

Risk avoidance or mitigation: The fifth pillar is risk avoidance or mitigation, which refers to essentially finding ways to eliminate or at least minimize risky behavior in one's life to the extent possible. General advice for self-care in this domain includes avoiding or quitting tobacco use, limiting or eliminating alcohol consumption, getting vaccinated, practicing safe sex, using sunscreen, not jumping off tall buildings (okay, that's just tongue-in-cheek), and so on. Basically, this pillar means avoiding behavior that is known to enhance risk to one's well-being in general.

Additionally, this pillar has particular implications for healthcare providers, given the nature of their work. We know that witnessing the death of another person is an inherently stressful and potentially severely traumatic experience. Physicians are, in many cases, exposed to this risk factor for stress, burnout, and PTSD. Mitigation of the risk associated with such situations includes minimizing exposure to them where possible. But where not possible, it's essential for organizations to provide mental health resources and for physicians to use them as needed (and help their peers access them as well). We will have more to say about the role of such counseling services later.

Good hygiene: Good hygiene refers to consistently performing the simple everyday tasks that we do to maintain cleanliness, physical well-being, and appearance, such as washing hands, brushing teeth, washing food before eating, and wearing clean clothes. In addition to acts promoting personal hygiene, we may consider such behaviors as cleaning our room, keeping the kitchen dishes from piling up, and engaging in other home-based hygienic practices as supporting overall hygiene. These behaviors are also essential in the workplace and are identified as a valuable a self-care strategy in that environment as well.

Rational and responsible use of products, services, diagnostics, and medicines: This pillar refers to being smart about the available products and services one uses, including diagnostic tools and medicines. That is, avoiding inappropriate use of prescription medicine is obvious, but so is being smart about over-the-counter products as well. In other words, following the labels on products and following recommended practices for available services (including mental health services) is essential to maintaining self-care. The human body is all too easily addicted to any number of substances and therefore care and attention is needed to bolster rather than undercut self-care aims.

Social self-care: In general, social support is widely acknowledged as one of the most critical stress-management, burnout mitigation, and longevity-promoting strategies available to us (e.g., Holt-Lunstad et al., 2010). It is such a crucially important, high-impact stress-management strategy that we devote all of the upcoming Chapter 7 to it. Here we touch on it briefly and introduce it as one of the identified pillars of strategic self-care. Briefly, social self-care refers to any and all actions that one takes to build and maintain positive social relationships with coworkers, close friends, and family. Such actions may include meeting up for a catch-up coffee, taking a break to meet for lunch, scheduling time on the weekend with friends to see a movie, or engaging in other nonwork activity. Social self-care also includes, critically, making time to bolster familial relationships, including time for a partner, children, and extended family. Family is a primary source of social support but is often a neglected domain when stress and burnout risks are mounting (Adams, King, & King, 1996). Ensuring adequate time to care for children, share moments with one's spouse or partner, and engage in mutually enjoyable activities together is essential to maintaining this critical reserve of social support.

Emotional self-care: Emotional self-care refers to activities that acknowledge the feelings one has related to both positive and negative experiences. Strategies for engaging in emotional self-care might include keeping a reflective journal (Wonders, 2018) and tracking how day-to-day emotional affect is going for you. That is, by tracking mood, one can see the patterns of ups and downs, and perhaps recognize the need for self-compassion (i.e., "Give yourself a break already!"). Becoming more mindful of one's mood in this way could help identify a string of days associated with negative emotions, setting off an automatic effort around self-care behaviors identified in the other pillars. Additionally, emotional self-care overlaps a bit with social self-care in that engaging in the reflective strategy often leads to conversations with others who can provide thoughts, guidance, ideas, and support.

Workplace self-care: Workplace self-care refers to activities designed to enhance one's ability to respond to stressful situations while at work (Selbst & Zultanky, 2020). For example, sometimes work-related situations are complex, difficult, and perhaps impossible to resolve alone. Thus, one strategy for enhancing resources to respond to challenging work situations is to identify a colleague who is trustworthy and who can be a sounding board, or who can even be a mentor. Again, the overlap with social support is evident in this example. Additionally, there are often environmental tools and resources at work that are intended to make work a bit more pleasant (e.g., the water cooler isn't there just to gather dust). Workplace self-care involves recognizing those provisions and using them. These provisions may include free-flowing coffee, or lunch and learn sessions, or even meditation opportunities (Lienke, 2021). Just because it's work does not mean that you aren't human and do not need to take a moment to care for your own needs, so you can care for others later. Companies consistently identified as "best places to work" generally provide these types of stress-reduction, pro-employee policies. Notable examples of such organizations in healthcare that endeavor to establish environments that enable workplace self-care include the Texas Institute for Surgery and the Chartis Group, among others (for a list, see Modern Healthcare, 2021).

Self-Care and Burnout among Physicians

As noted, some of the pillars will seem obviously intuitive for physicians and other healthcare providers. However, some of the pillars and the strategies that support them are not as intuitive, or perhaps we are just less inclined to follow them. This section and the remaining sections will focus more on what we know from science concerning the importance of self-care specifically for physicians and healthcare workers. The bottom line is that while self-care matters and is a good thing for *all* people, of course, it is especially critical for physicians who are at risk for burnout, with all its negative effects on themselves and their patients.

To begin, a surprisingly large amount of self-care research was published in 2020, focused on understanding how self-care impacts on-the-job behavior. For example, Shanafelt and colleagues (2020) investigated the relationship between the self-care practices of physician leaders and their independently assessed leadership behavior. Much to our surprise, none of the ten pillars identified by other authors and consolidated by us in this chapter addresses the self-care topic in the Shanafelt et al. (2020) study, namely, sleep. Interestingly, these authors found that sleep-related impairment in physician leaders was positively related to sleep-related impairment among their subordinates. To extrapolate from this finding, leaders' examples of self-care may make others in their group more or less likely to engage in self-care. Further, their study showed that as self-care increased, perceived leadership effectiveness increased. Thus, as we know, leaders' behavior influences how others behave in general, and in this specific case the behavior that was modeled was self-care in the form of sleep.

The Special Case for Sleep

Given what Shanafelt and colleagues (2020) showed in the study referenced above, we decided to take a closer look at self-care and sleep. In a related study, Stewart and colleagues (2019) also focused on the issue of sleep and burnout. Essentially, occupational and personal health play a substantial role in physician burnout, including the fact that sleep deprivation is all too common among physicians. The link between sleep deprivation and burnout has been shown in studies with a variety of workers across industries. Nearly half (43 percent) of physicians acknowledge that sleep loss is tied to their work schedule (American College of Chest Physicians, 2008).

There are several research-based models that describe the relationship between burnout and sleep. Most suggest a potential causal mechanism between sleep disturbance and burnout (Stewart et al., 2019). Sleep deprivation leads to a chronic depletion of energy stores and activation of the hypothalamic-pituitary-adrenal axis, thereby increasing levels of bodily physical stress response. Thus, if the work cycles and schedules for physicians make a good number of them sleep deprived, it translates rather quickly to high burnout risk overall. Overall, the evidence clearly suggests that many physicians experience sleep deprivation, and so do nurses, medical students, and residents.

Thus, Stewart and colleagues (2019) recommend early detection and intervention to reduce sleep deprivation among healthcare workers. Interventions for healthy sleep practices begin with the physician, though we also recommend that adjustments are made to the healthcare system, which we discuss further in Chapter 14. The implementation of healthy sleep practices begins with clinicians. Good sleep practices include simply seeking adequate sleep, with strategies such as going to bed when tired and not before, setting a fixed wake time, avoiding naps, and always avoiding drowsy driving (Consensus Conference Panel, 2015). Physicians also need greater control of work time, which is an important determinant of reduced workplace stress and which can diminish the negative impact on sleep quality of long or night shifts (Tucker et al., 2015). Again, this is a systems issue to which we will return.

A Look at Mindfulness and Self-Compassion

The good news about self-care and burnout is there are many constructive self-care habits that can be learned and implemented that mitigate burnout. Sleep matters greatly, and we hope that physicians are able to address that issue to some extent themselves with the sorts of strategies outlined above. However, in addition to sleep-improvement strategies, Kemper and colleagues (2015) investigated two trainable practices, namely, mindfulness and self-compassion, which could potentially enhance resilience and mitigate burnout. Similar to the ninth pillar, mindfulness has been defined as paying attention to the present moment in a particularly nonjudgmental way (Ockene, Ockene, Kabat-Zinn, Greene, & Frid, 1990). Mindfulness training appears to be related to reductions in burnout and also to increases in empathy in a variety of work settings (Kabat-Zinn & Hanh, 2009). Self-compassion refers to being kind to oneself as one would to others, and recognizing of one's common humanity with others (Neff, 2003). It differs from mindfulness in that the focus is not on a specific moment but on situations in general that an individual experiences.

Although others have shown the usefulness of training in these concepts in reducing burnout in other industries, Kemper et al. (2015) wanted to study the effect on physicians. Their results indicated that mindfulness and self-compassion were both strongly related to resilience in a positive way, thereby having the potential to reduce burnout. These findings suggest that when organizations offer training in mindfulness or self-compassion, healthcare workers may very well want to enroll and engage.

Summing Up

Of the many strategies for minimizing the negative effects of stress, the self-care strategies are among the easiest to implement, as they are largely under the control of the individual. It doesn't take any major systems-level or teams-level change for individuals to recognize the value of rest, diet, and exercise in promoting their overall health and reducing their risk of burnout. As much as doctors and other healthcare providers preach these strategies to their patients, appropriately, many in the healthcare enterprise do not always follow their own advice. As important as it is to the individual to practice health-promoting behaviors consistent with these strategies, it is also important to their coworkers. Research shows that the specific behaviors of leaders (in healthcare and in other settings) strongly influence the behaviors of others with whom they work.

The COVID-19 Effect

The ongoing pandemic puts a premium on any and all stress-management strategies. As the self-care strategies are widely recognized as comparatively easy to implement, and largely though not entirely under the control of the individual, they should be used by healthcare workers at all levels. Recognizing that there are other beneficial strategies, we should also recognize the significant stress-buffering effect of strengthening body and mind in order to offset the deleterious effects of excessive stress.

Key Takeaways

- In addition to better understand one's own personality and possible associated risk factors for burnout and strategies to reduce that risk, it is helpful for individuals to attend to self-care.

- Self-care strategies are for the most part more easily implemented than personality traits. They are more directly under the control of the individual.
- Specifically, individuals can get more rest. They may not be able to "will themselves to sleep," but they can take time away from work, disengage from their work-related stressors, and spend more time relaxing. Additionally, there are promising data to support the use of meditation techniques, not only to help the individual relax during the meditative state but also to be better able to relax (even to sleep) in the long term.
- A healthy diet and moderate exercise are universally recommended as self-care/stress management strategies.
- It is useful for physicians and other leaders in healthcare to recognize the extent to which their self-care behaviors influence the self-care behaviors of their coworkers.
- The continuing COVID crisis calls for everyone, definitely including physicians and other healthcare providers, to implement every possible stress-control strategy. The bundle of strategies summarized as self-care strategies, and under the control of the individual, are relatively easily implemented. They should be a focal point for doctors.

REFERENCES

Adams, G. A., King, L. A., & King, D. W. (1996). Relationships of job and family involvement, family social support, and work–family conflict with job and life satisfaction. *Journal of Applied Psychology, 81*(4), 411.

American College of Chest Physicians. (2008, March 5). Most physicians sleep fewer hours than needed for peak performance, report says. *ScienceDaily.* Retrieved June 30, 2021, from www.sciencedaily.com/releases/2008/03/080304075723.htm.

Consensus Conference Panel, Watson, N. F., Badr, M. S., Belenky, G., Bliwise, D. L., Buxton, O. M., Buysse, D., Dinges, D. F., Gangwisch, J., Grandner, M. A., Kushida, C., Malhotra, R. K., Martin, J. L., Patel, S. R., Quan, S. F., & Tasali, E. (2015). Joint consensus statement of the American Academy of Sleep Medicine and Sleep Research Society on the recommended amount of sleep for a healthy adult: Methodology and discussion. *Sleep, 38*(8), 1161–1183. https://doi.org/10.5665/sleep.4886.

Holt-Lunstad, J., Smith, T. B., & Layton, J. B. (2010). Social relationships and mortality risk: A meta-analytic review. *PLoS Medicine, 7*(7), 1–20.

ISF. (2020, November 17). About ISF. https://isfglobal.org/about-isf/.

Kabat-Zinn, J., & Hanh, T. N. (2009). *Full Catastrophe Living: Using the Wisdom of Your Body and Mind to Face Stress, Pain, and Illness.* McHenry, IL: Delta.

Kemper, K. J., Mo, X., & Khayat, R. (2015). Are mindfulness and self-compassion associated with sleep and resilience in health professionals? *The Journal of Alternative and Complementary Medicine, 21*(8), 496–503.

Klaperski, S., Koch, E., Hewel, D., Schempp, A., & Müller, J. (2019). Optimizing mental health benefits of exercise: The influence of the exercise environment on acute stress levels and wellbeing. *Mental Health & Prevention, 15*, 173–200.

Lienke, C. B. (2021, June 1). How to meditate at work: launch a regular meditation practice. FlexJobs. www.flexjobs.com/blog/post/how-to-medi tate-at-work/#:~:text=Whether%20youre%20working%20at,your%20atten-tion%20span%20and%20health.&text=Additionally%2C%20researchers%20have%20found%20that,reduce%20stress%20levels%20by%2040%25.

Modern Healthcare. (2021, May 15). Best places to work in healthcare: 2021 (alphabetical list). Modern Healthcare. www.modernhealthcare.com/labor/best-places-work-healthcare-2021-alphabetical-list.

Neff, K. D. (2003). The development and validation of a scale to measure self-compassion. *Self and Identity, 2*(3), 223–250.

Ockene, J. K., Ockene, I. S., Kabat-Zinn, J., Greene, H. L., & Frid, D. (1990). Teaching risk-factor counseling skills to medical students, house staff, and fellows. *American Journal of Preventive Medicine, 6*(2 Suppl), 35–42.

Selbst, M., & Zultanky, A. (2020). Managing burnout and compassion fatigue through self-care strategies. Behavior Therapy Associates. https://behaviortherapyassociates.com/act/managing-burnout-and-compassion-fatigue-through-self-care-strategies/.

Shanafelt, T. D., Makowski, M. S., Wang, H., Bohman, B., Leonard, M., Harrington, R. A., ... & Trockel, M. (2020). Association of burnout, professional fulfillment, and self-care practices of physician leaders with their independently rated leadership effectiveness. *JAMA Network Open, 3*(6), e207961–e207961.

Stewart, N. H., & Arora, V. M. (2019). The impact of sleep and circadian disorders on physician burnout. *Chest, 156*(5), 1022–1030.

Tucker, P., Bejerot, E., Kecklund, G., Aronsson, G., & Åkerstedt, T. (2015). The impact of work time control on physicians' sleep and well-being. *Applied Ergonomics, 47*, 109–116. https://doi.org/10.1016/j.apergo.2014.09.001.

Wonders, L. (2018, July 10). Avoiding burnout: 10 tips for self-care. Wonders Counseling Services. https://wonderscounseling.com/burnout/.

World Health Organization. (1998). The role of the pharmacist in self-care and self-medication: Report of the 4th WHO Consultative Group on the Role of the Pharmacist, The Hague, Netherlands, August 26–28, 1998.

CHAPTER 7

Solution #3: Seek Social Support

After a particularly hard shift where several patients passed from complications with COVID, a friend of mine walked up to me and said, "You're the only reason I don't quit this f-ing job."
—Charge nurse

When difficult things happen, when challenging situations arise, we often reach out to a colleague or friend for thoughts, guidance, and insight, or just a chance to talk it out. This strategy of seeking and using social support, touched on briefly in earlier chapters, is sufficiently powerful, even critical, that it deserves its own chapter. Recently, Joe found himself in such a challenging and stressful situation. As a professor, challenging circumstances can range from a difficult boss to uncooperative colleagues, problematic students, and beyond. Replace students with customers or patients, and most readers of this book can relate. What did he do? He contacted a colleague at another institution and vented, seeking external social support from a trusted source. It may come as no surprise that, while personality-based and self-care strategies are important components of a comprehensive strategy, the stress-management literature consistently points to social support (such as seeking out advice from a colleague like Joe did) as not only an important strategy, but arguably the single most effective individual strategy to manage stress.

According to the American Psychological Association, social support is "the provision of assistance or comfort to others, typically to help them cope with biological, psychological, and social stressors" (APA, 2020). Note the emphasis, appropriately, on "stressors." This form of support can come from any interpersonal relation in a person's social or work network. Individuals who can provide social support include, but are not limited to, family members, neighbors, friends, caregivers, colleagues at work, support groups, and religious institutions. The nature of the support can be very practical in nature, such as assisting with chores at home

(reducing workload), offering advice (giving fresh ideas), or simply providing an opportunity to "get it off your chest," as Joe's colleague did.
What's critical is that the social support individual or group be completely
trusted. Seeking help and talking about one's stresses make one vulnerable.
That is not a concern if the support person or group provides psychological
safety, allowing the individual under stress to be open and honest, without
prejudice. While we typically picture social support being practical in the
sense outlined above, it can also take the form of material or tangible
assistance, such as money or other resources. Parents provide that form of
social support to their children, particularly older children as they "leave
the nest" and seek to get further education, purchase a home, and so on.
But the social support that Joe sought and used was more reflective of
emotional concern that helped him feel valued, accepted, and understood.

Types of Social Support

Given the varied nature of social support, it probably comes as no surprise
that at least four types of social support have been identified in the research
literature (Jacobson, 1986). We discuss each type here and provide examples from healthcare environments, as a way for our readers to begin to
identify them in their own experiences. While we discuss the four types
separately for purposes of analysis, in fact, actual expressions of social
support most often combine two or more of the four types.

The first type of social support is emotional support (Heaney & Israel,
2008). Emotional support includes expressions of empathy, love, understanding, trust, and care. In other words, it is what Joe sought from his
colleague. Close friends, family members, and valued colleagues are likely
individuals who can provide a listening ear. For physicians and healthcare
workers, such emotional support would be especially valuable, for example,
when a particularly difficult patient interaction occurs. Perhaps the patient is
being difficult, or perhaps the disease is more aggressive than first thought,
or perhaps the patient reminds you of a loved one, which causes stronger
empathic feeling. Emotional support in this case is having someone nearby,
another physician or healthcare worker, who will listen to the concerns or
feelings and perhaps provide both empathy and understanding.

The second type of social support is instrumental support (Shakespeare-
Finch & Obst, 2011). This form of support is the tangible aid or service
that is rendered at a moment's notice, often in a time of crisis. We are
guessing that many of our readers are immediately thinking of a time in

recent months, during the COVID-19 pandemic, when a colleague provided tangible, immediate, instrumental support. For example, perhaps one's PPE started to fall off at a particularly vulnerable moment (e.g., emergency room physician assisting with a bed transfer), and a colleague stepped in. Perhaps the tangible support comes outside the working situation, when colleagues assist each other with transportation of their children to or from the daycare near their homes. Again, the idea here is that someone is in need and tangible support is provided.

Informational support is the third identified type of support (Langford et al., 1997). Informational support is advice, information, and suggestions related to the problem, challenge, or concern that required the support. Probably as no surprise, emotional and informational support often coincide. After all, when a friend comes looking for support, we often both empathize and give them an idea of what they could do, perhaps based on a story or experience from our past. Imagine someone coming to a peer physician to discuss a patient who is noncompliant with their care plan, and all their friend says is, "Oh gosh, I'm so sorry. That must be really tough. I understand how you feel. There, there." Frankly, we would probably feel like that's pretty crappy support and seek another colleague for advice, suggestions on how to fix the problem. Thus, it is common for emotional support to be followed by another form of support, either informational or instrumental advice (Lloyd-Jones, 2021). Note too, though, that sometimes people do mainly want to vent and don't want someone to "tell them what to do." Balance is critical here.

The fourth type of social support is called appraisal support (Heaney & Israel, 2008). Sometimes referred to as reappraisal, appraisal support is the act of using available information to properly assess and evaluate or reevaluate the situation (Lazarus, 1995). Essentially, this is reframing the situation as more manageable by obtaining more accurate information about the challenge, or the best way to respond to or deal with the situation. Such an appraisal can result in a socially constructed reality allowing for the appropriate management of the situation, minimizing the stress. For example, perhaps the day starts with a physician realizing, once again, they are so overbooked that they may not be able to find time for a restroom break until after what will likely be a missed lunch break. Appraisal, or in this case reappraisal (taking information that person already has and helping them see it in a different light), occurs when a fellow physician or other healthcare worker provides information (e.g., one upcoming appointment will be a short procedure) that changes the nature of the original situation. Thus, reappraisal is a specific form, a subtype of informational support. Rather than tell you what to do, the colleague who is offering appraisal support is really saying, "Think about it this way instead."

Social Support and Physician Burnout

Equipped with a more detailed understanding of what social support looks like, we now turn our attention to the research that squarely places it as a key and meaningful resource to reduce, and in some cases potentially eliminate, burnout among physicians and healthcare workers (Hamama et al., 2019). In other words, what does social support specifically look and sound like for physicians and other healthcare workers?

An interesting starting point comes from the work of Rogers and colleagues (2016) concerning burnout among physician residents. Specifically, they asked the residents about their friend-based and colleague-based support, their perceived loneliness, and their levels of personal and work-related burnout. They hypothesized that social support would reduce burnout, but primarily by reducing loneliness. Their analyses showed that the more support a resident felt from their friends and colleagues, the less they felt lonely, and the lower their reported levels of burnout. It may come as no surprise given the context that nonwork friend support appeared to have a slightly stronger relationship with both loneliness and burnout when compared to colleague support. But of course that is not to minimize the importance of colleague support.

In 2019, Hamama and colleagues published a study of nurses' and physicians' burnout as potentially impacted by perceived social support. Their interest was in assessing whether social support would reduce secondary traumatic stress and the subsequent resulting burnout. Secondary traumatic stress is a form of stress caused by witnessing traumatic events occurring to others. The study results indicated that perceived social support reduced both the experience of secondary traumatic stress and burnout among nurses and physicians, with the effect being stronger for nurses.

There are many, many other studies linking social support and burnout (e.g., Ma et al., 2020; Zhang et al., 2020), with the bottom line being that social support consistently, across a variety of healthcare contexts, appears to reduce the overall risk of burnout. Let's explore social support a bit further, focusing on optimal ways of giving and receiving social support. Specifically, let's look at the critical social norm of reciprocity.

How Physicians Give and Get Social Support to Reduce Burnout

Because social support comes from those within our personal and professional network, the key to both getting and giving social support to others is building and maintaining that network. In order to do that, one must fully embrace the norm of reciprocity (Lu, 1997). Reciprocity refers to the practice of exchanging things with others for mutual benefit. The norm of reciprocity means that within certain cultures (including organizational cultures), it is normative or common for reciprocity to be expected and to occur. In a culture that values reciprocity, physicians and healthcare workers who give social support, in all the forms outlined previously, are more likely to receive social support in their own time of need. That's how it works.

Barriers to Social Support

There are several common barriers to implementing this healthy and effective strategy of social support. The personality variables discussed earlier impact individuals' willingness and ability to talk it out. First, positive, optimistic, confident individuals are not always the best judge of when they are "in too deep." Their very internal locus of control, high self-efficacy, and tendency to use constructive self-talk can mire them into thinking they can go it alone, that they will be okay no matter what. While such attitudes are generally healthy and beneficial, when the stress reaches a certain level, no amount of individual self-sufficiency can take care of it. Also, it is common for confident people not to want to "burden" others with their problems. And critically, competent and confident people generally don't want to appear "weak and needy."

All of the aforementioned barriers apply as well, and perhaps more strongly for Type A individuals. Also, research has suggested that Type As, by virtue of their competitiveness (and possibly anger-hostility), may not generally have the kinds of support systems that others enjoy. And they may be most reluctant to reach out to others for help. Recall how common the hard-charging, competitive, achievement-oriented Type A personality is among physicians (hopefully without the toxic anger-hostility axis).

Reaching out for social support is an act of vulnerability. It is a statement of "I need help." Given their personality and the requirements of the role they are in, doctors and other healthcare workers may well find it hard to "confess weakness," as that is how it may appear to them. Do they tell their boss or coworkers that they are struggling? What is critical for social support to be sought and given is that there be a high level of trust between the individuals who seek and give social support. None of the potential value of social support is realized if the relationship is not completely trusted. We cannot overemphasize the importance of the trust factor.

Employee Assistance Programs

While we will talk about employee assistance programs (EAPs) in more detail later as an element of systems solutions, for now note that the role that EAP counselors play is exactly that of a trusted colleague/friend who will provide emotional support, possibly instrumental support, and definitely informational and reappraisal support. Many hospital systems provide EAP options to their staff, especially as the burnout crisis has become so visible in recent times. But again, the challenge is for doctors and others to be trusting in the confidentiality of the counseling relationship and willing to use the institutional social support that is available to them. The data so far suggest that EAPs are underutilized.

Summing Up

Social support is consistently identified in the stress-management literature going back many decades as a primary individual strategy for reducing stress. Talking it out with trusted family members, colleagues, and friends can provide emotional support, tangible instrumental support, informational support, and reappraisal support, all of which add up to lowering the risk of burnout. And like the other individual strategies discussed here, it is under the control of the individual. The challenge is getting hard-charging, achievement-oriented, self-confident individuals to accept the value in seeking and getting social support, and then to implement that strategy as a central part of their stress-management, burnout-reduction strategy.

The COVID-19 Effect

Research consistently shows that social support is the single most effective stress-management strategy, and as the pandemic has so dramatically spiked the stress level of all in healthcare, the focus on social support becomes that much more critical. As much as overworked frontline healthcare providers may feel they don't have the time to "sit down and talk it out" with family, friends, or colleagues and/or don't want to burden them, it is now more critical than ever to acknowledge and use social support as a primary buffer to the stress reaction. It is our hope that any stigma connected with "going to the EAP" is reduced in these most trying times.

Key Takeaways

- Social support is a highly effective individual stress-management strategy that is widely identified as critical in reducing burnout risk.
- The four major types of social support are identified as emotional, instrumental, informational, and reappraisal.
- In most cases a social support interaction will comprise several of the types. A trusted colleague, friend, or family member may express empathy, offer tangible help or advice, and/or frame ways of "seeing it differently."
- Physicians and other healthcare workers are likely to underutilize informal or structured (e.g., employee assistance programs) social support, feeling that they should be strong enough to handle things on their own and not wanting to "burden" others with their problems.

REFERENCES

APA. (2020). Social support. APA Dictionary of Psychology. https://dictionary .apa.org/social-support.

Hamama, L., Hamama-Raz, Y., Stokar, Y. N., Pat-Horenczyk, R., Brom, D., & Bron-Harlev, E. (2019). Burnout and perceived social support: The mediating role of secondary traumatization in nurses vs. physicians. *Journal of Advanced Nursing*, 75(11), 2742–2752. https://doi.org/10.1111/jan.14122.

Heaney, C. A., & Israel, B. A. (2008). Social networks and social support. In *Health Behavior and Health Education: Theory, Research, and Practice*, 4th ed., ed. K. Glanz, B. K. Rimer, & K. Viswanath (pp. 189–210). Jossey-Bass.

Jacobson D. E. (1986). Types and timing of social support. *Journal of Health and Social Behavior*, 27(3), 250–264.

Langford, C. P., Bowsher, J., Maloney, J. P., & Lillis, P. P. (1997). Social support: A conceptual analysis. *Journal of Advanced Nursing*, 25(1), 95–100. https://doi.org/10.1046/j.1365-2648.1997.1997025095.x.

Lazarus, R. S. (1995). Vexing research problems inherent in cognitive-mediational theories of emotion – and some solutions. *Psychological Inquiry*, 6(3), 183–196.

Lloyd-Jones, B. (2021). Developing competencies for emotional, instrumental, and informational student support during the COVID-19 pandemic:

A human relations/human resource development approach. *Advances in Developing Human Resources, 23*(1), 41–54.

Lu, L. (1997). Social support, reciprocity, and well-being. *The Journal of Social Psychology, 137*(5), 618–628.

Ma, H., Qiao, H., Qu, H., Wang, H., Huang, Y., Cheng, H., . . . & Zhang, N. (2020). Role stress, social support and occupational burnout among physicians in China: A path analysis approach. *International Health, 12*(3), 157–163.

Rogers, E., Polonijo, A. N., & Carpiano, R. M. (2016). Getting by with a little help from friends and colleagues: Testing how residents' social support networks affect loneliness and burnout. *Canadian Family Physician/ Medecin de famille canadien, 62*(11), e677–e683.

Shakespeare-Finch, J., & Obst, P. L. (2011). The development of the 2-Way Social Support Scale: A measure of giving and receiving emotional and instrumental support. *Journal of Personality Assessment, 93*(5), 483–490. https://doi.org/10.1080/00223891.2011.594124.

Zhang, H., Ye, Z., Tang, L., Zou, P., Du, C., Shao, J., . . . & Mu, S. Y. (2020). Anxiety symptoms and burnout among Chinese medical staff of intensive care unit: The moderating effect of social support. *BMC Psychiatry, 20*, 1–7.

CHAPTER 8

Solution #4: Follow the Advice You Would Give Patients

> I just looked in the mirror one day, wasn't happy with what I saw,
> and realized I was a hypocrite who didn't follow the Hippocratic
> Oath for myself. It was time to make a change and so I did.
>
> —Family physician

The previous three solutions that we proposed were individual-focused, and with the exception of radically changing one's personality instead of developing work-arounds, for the most part are actionable right now. The fourth solution discussed here is also under the control of the individual and thus highly actionable, but does not provide new strategies beyond the first three. The fourth solution is to follow the advice that physicians or healthcare workers (such as you might be) give patients relative to managing their mental, emotional, and physical health in dealing with the stresses in their lives. Too often physicians and medical providers operate under the venerable phrase, "Do as I say, not as I do." Parents often fall into this trap with their children, as do consultants with the organizations they work with, counselors with their clients, and so physicians with their patients. In this chapter, rather than introducing new individual-level actions to take, we discuss possible reasons that physicians and healthcare providers so often do not take their own sage advice. Obviously, we encourage them to do so.

The Physician Risk Taker

In an interesting study of physicians' reactions to hypothetical treatment scenarios (Reuters Life!, 2011), a comparison was made between physicians and (nonphysician) patients. Physicians were given hypothetical scenarios in which they were a sick person with a few different therapies to choose from. The therapies came with more or fewer side effects, and some were much riskier in terms of possible fatal consequences than others. Ultimately, physicians chose therapies that had higher risk of death, but fewer severe side effects. In other words, they made the risker choice, compared to nonphysicians. In most cases, one would assume that a physician would encourage their patients to be risk averse as it pertains to their lives, and yet they seem less risk averse with their own. This seemingly risky attitude plays out in more mundane decisions as well.

As we noted earlier, John's wife is a retired nurse, and he has heard her say on more than a few occasions, "Doctors and nurses are the worst patients." A physician that she sees at least annually is a dear friend and wonderful doctor who is overweight and a (former) heavy smoker. It is not likely that this excellent physician would tell his patients, "I recommend you pack on about twenty-five pounds and start smoking." *Knowledge does not change behavior.*

Psychologists often study decision making and try to understand why humans so often tend to do the opposite of what they know to be right, to be less risky or dangerous, and why they sometimes do what is downright stupid, even when they know (or at least later acknowledge) it is downright stupid. For example, a study of firefighters (Maglio et al., 2016) found that fewer than 50 percent of firefighters choose to wear their critical personal protective equipment (PPE) during situations known to expose firefighters to carcinogens, even though their training clearly indicated that they should. One reason for the disconnect between knowledge and behavior is the pressures within an industry and within society at large. Quoting a firefighter from Maglio and colleagues' study: "Our society still has a romanticized notion of what firefighters do, which is kill themselves. And we do everything we can in the fire service to reinforce that." Another followed that up by saying, "We're firemen, we don't like to be known as being overly safe, I guess." With occupational identity of that nature, reinforced by a society that idolizes the hero firefighter, it's no wonder that they do not always put on their required PPE.

In a similar vein, we have talked with highly experienced factory workers about their approach to safe work, and have often heard, "I have been doing this for many years.... I know what to touch and what not to touch.... I will teach new-hires 'by the book,' but in all honesty, I do take short-cuts.... It's automatic for me now." As we noted earlier, industrial accidents are surprisingly common even among the most experienced workers, often especially among those experienced workers. Having sat in on countless accident investigations, we have never heard an experienced worker who suffered an injury say, "I didn't know the proper procedure.... I wasn't trained.... I wasn't sure whether I was supposed to use PPE." To the contrary, we have most often heard, "I knew better.... I just got in a hurry ... took a shortcut.... It was stupid.... I should have locked out power to that saw."

The disconnect between safety knowledge and safe behavior, known as the "black box of decision-making" (Maglio et al., 2016), is definitely present among physicians. For example, a Dr. Montgomery in an interview with *Time* magazine stated, "It's unrealistic to expect that knowledge should prompt physicians to avoid unhealthy behaviors.... Just like everybody else, they have a low risk perception with regard to their health" (Sifferlin, 2014). The idea that "it can't happen to me" is not just a patient phenomenon, but also a provider or physician concern, because they too are human.

In fact, the onset of bad health behaviors usually occurs early on for physicians, even during medical school, and continuing thereafter. For example, fifty years ago, it was not uncommon to see a physician or nurse taking smoke breaks. Print ads for cigarettes years ago often featured physicians touting the brand they smoked and/or the brand they recommended to their patients. Over time, the prevalence of smoking among healthcare providers has reduced, just as it has in the general population (Sifferlin, 2014), but not to zero.

In an effort to begin to work on this issue of "Do as I say, not as I do," about a decade ago a couple of medical students proposed "The Patient Promise" (Lu, 2012). One of these students, Shiv Gaglani, said, "We realized that many of the harmful lifestyle behaviors we were learning to counsel against as future physicians were actually becoming part of our daily lives" (Sifferlin, 2014). Medical school stress was leading him and his peers to eat less healthily, sleep much less, exercise more infrequently if at all, and engage in other lifestyle behaviors in order to cope that would not be advised to most patients. In fact, another physician recently stated the following:

> We should strive to be the best versions of ourselves always, but also recognize that we are not above the maladies that may afflict our patients. If a patient states they are struggling with work and feel they need to drink more lately, it is okay to recognize that you as a doctor have experienced that problem too. When you advise your patient to cut back on the booze, take a day off work, and get better, remember that can be an option for you as well. (Morgan, 2017)

In other words, from medical school to the patient bedside, physicians in training and in practice need to practice what they preach.

The Data and the Ask

Let's look at the most current data as of this writing, as shown in Figure 8.1 (Kane, 2020). As we do, it should be noted that several of these statistics were reported in previous chapters, reported in the article by Leslie Kane summarizing a Medscape survey, and we now pull them together here in a central place to emphasize our point.

Paradoxically, in the social support category the isolation strategy was chosen by respondents nearly as often as the talk-it-out strategy. Questions remain as to whether these were the same respondents who alternately choose both strategies, or if different doctors responded differently. Regardless, it is unlikely that any doctor would recommend to their patients who are struggling with stress to isolate themselves, eat junk food, drink alcohol, and/or binge eat. But, as stated and discussed earlier, that's what many of them say they do, by their own admission.

How do doctors handle stress?

According to the 2020 Medscape survey of more than 15,000 doctors in the U.S., these strategies were used to handle stress:

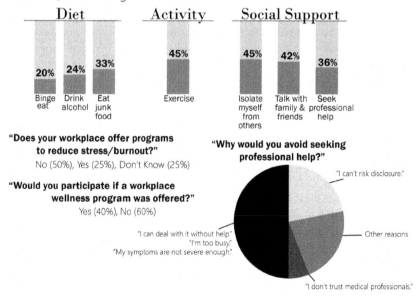

Figure 8.1　How do doctors handle stress?

Solution #4 is pretty simple. Physicians need to do the things that they prescribe for their patients facing similar stressful, burnout-prone situations. However, taking one's own advice is not easy for most people. For example, let's start with rest and relaxation. For a variety of systems reasons that we will explore later, doctors are typically working long hours over many consecutive weeks or even months, which makes the prospect of taking any vacation time off challenging – not to mention the barrier that these long work hours present to getting daily adequate rest. Of course, it is important to understand one critical (albeit obvious) fact about sleep. It's not something that can simply be *done*. Sleep can be attempted but an individual may not succeed. Ironically, one of the side effects of burnout is insomnia. As much as adequate rest is an identified self-care strategy that is critical to stress management, stress makes it harder to get adequate sleep, even with the strategies suggested in Chapter 6.

Similarly, an individual can have the best intentions in terms of eating better, exercising more, and talking out issues with others, but fail at all of them. A busy work schedule can lead to a lack of time to prepare and eat nutritious meals. Similarly, exercise – essential as it is – takes time away from work. Can most doctors afford thirty to forty minutes of vigorous physical activity per day? And, of course, talking it out is something doctors *can* do, but intention does not equal action for reasons we just discussed.

If you are thinking we seem to be repeating ourselves here as we explain our proposed solution #4, that's because we strongly recommend engaging in solutions #1, #2, and #3. They just happen to be the very things that physicians and medical providers tell most of the patients. It has been and remains very good advice.

Summing Up

The data point clearly in the direction of unhealthy habits and risky behaviors on the part of healthcare providers, contrary to the advice they universally give their patients. Such dysfunctional behaviors are exacerbated by stress and are often ineffective attempts at coping. The bottom line is that doctors and other healthcare providers should listen to themselves and follow their own advice.

The COVID-19 Effect

Simply put, the added stress of the pandemic makes it that much more critical that doctors adhere to a rational stress-management strategy that includes all the individual strategies they invariably advise their patients to follow.

Key Takeaways

- Doctors are great at giving good healthcare advice in general, and in particular regarding stress management. They are not so good at following their own good advice.
- Especially during times of additional stress for all, it is more critical than ever that healthcare providers do what they counsel their patients to do.

REFERENCES

Dow Jones & Company. (2014, August 11). What is the most common piece of advice doctors give – but don't take? *Wall Street Journal.* www.wsj.com/articles/what-is-the-most-common-piece-of-advice-doctors-givebut-dont-take-1407760460.

Kane, L. (2020, January 15). Medscape National Physician Burnout & Suicide Report 2020: The generational divide. Medscape.com. www.medscape.com/slideshow/2020-lifestyle-burnout-6012460?faf=1.

Lu, S. (2012, October 25). The patient promise: Healers pledge to lead by example. TEDMED Blog. https://blog.tedmed.com/the-patient-promise-doctors-pledge-to-lead-by-example/.

Maglio, M. A., Scott, C., Davis, A. L., Allen, J., & Taylor, J. A. (2016). Situational pressures that influence firefighters' decision making about personal protective equipment: A qualitative analysis. *American Journal of Health Behavior, 40*(5), 555–567.

Morgan, J. C. (2017, March 6). Doctors don't often follow their own advice. KevinMD.com. www.kevinmd.com/blog/2017/03/doctors-dont-often-follow-advice.html.

Reuters Life! (2011, April 12). Doctors don't always take their own advice: Survey. Reuters. www.reuters.com/article/us-doctors-advice-life/doctors-dont-always-take-their-own-advice-survey-idUSTRE73B0IZ20110412.

Sifferlin, A. (2014, September 23). When doctors ignore their own advice. *Time.* https://time.com/3421538/doctors-ignore-advice/.

CHAPTER 9

Solution #5: Perform Effective Team Leadership

> When I think of my clinic, my colleagues, my nurses, and my admin personnel, we really are a team.... I mean it's kind of like we're team-based medical practice.
>
> —Family physician

Although individual efforts are essential to reducing burnout, and are most under the control of the individual, those efforts can get a person only so far. Thus, this chapter and the next two focus on the team setting and on teamwork strategies that help in reducing the risk of burnout. In healthcare, many physicians work in groups or networks of colleagues who interact, share patients, give referrals, and provide team care for their patients. The team setting where physicians interact is the next level at which stress-management solutions can and should be situated. Although there is an extensive body of literature in the social and behavioral science on groups and teams in general, there is a smaller but growing body of literature on teams in healthcare specifically, including the crucial aspects of team leadership, team collaborative processes, and overall team culture. Our team-based solutions tackle each of these three general domains of teamwork in turn, with the current chapter focused on effective team leadership. Chapter 10 then addresses the issue of peer-level collaboration in teams, and Chapter 11 discusses the importance of establishing and maintaining an overall positive team culture and provides higher-order strategies for doing so. In each case, we define the domain and discuss what it looks like in the healthcare environment based on the existing literature, our interviews, and our own observations. Then we describe how we can leverage the resources of the team to reduce burnout experienced by physicians and others in the healthcare environment. Before focusing on team leadership, let's look at what the research literature says about leadership and leadership styles in general.

Leadership and Leadership Styles

Leaders inspire, encourage, and support others (their followers) in working toward a common goal (Gentry, 2016). In exerting their leadership, they may demonstrate any of several primary styles that have been identified in the literature on leadership. What are those styles?

Many decades of research have shown that there are different types of leaders with distinctively different prevailing styles of leadership. Rather than attempt to present an exhaustive list here, we will focus our discussion on three primary types that have been much researched and are prominent in the contemporary leadership literature, namely, charismatic leadership, transformational leadership, and laissez-faire leadership (Judge et al., 2006). In discussing them, it will quickly become clear which leadership styles are associated with reduced burnout and which are more likely to create an environment in which burnout will emerge for the leader and their followers on their team.

The first type we discuss here is charismatic leadership. "Charisma" refers to "compelling attractiveness or charm that can inspire devotion in others" (Oxford Advanced Learner's Dictionary). Thus, a charismatic leader is inspiring, well liked, and expressive in their communication and demeanor, such that people desire to follow them and remain connected to them (Gentry, 2016). The earliest leadership researchers considered charisma to be the superpower of charismatic leaders, and to be the primary way in which they derive their authority (Weber, 1947). Further, House (1976) and Judge and colleagues (2006) identified several key behaviors associated with charismatic leadership. Charismatic leaders maintain a strong vision for the future, tend to be risk takers in their efforts to enact their vision, are sensitive to their followers' needs, and are both competent and knowledgeable about what they are trying to achieve. Because such leaders are driven by their values and aims, and their values and aims can be negative as well as positive, charismatic leadership is not always associated with what society would identify as good outcomes. At moderate levels of manifestation among leaders, charismatic leadership can enable great progress toward goals while maintaining follower health and well-being. However, the risk-taking willingness and the drive to achieve can overpower the more altruistic goals and can, in the more extreme cases, create an environment that does not support health and well-being, but which sacrifices those aims in order to achieve the superordinate goal. And note that the overall effect of charismatic leadership not only depends on the strength of the characteristic; it also depends critically on the nature of the vision that is driving the leader's behavior.

Some widely cited examples of charismatic leaders in recent history include Martin Luther King Jr., Margaret Thatcher, and Jack Welch (McManus, 2021). These individuals exemplify all we've mentioned so far concerning charismatic leaders. Still, exceptionally charismatic leaders may also become overly confident and create a level of dependence on them that inhibits succession planning, ultimately resulting in a leadership crisis (Yukl, 2010). Some believe that former founder/CEO of Apple, Steve Jobs, was an example of such a leader (Nguyen, 2017). Although Tim Cook has certainly done well enough for the Apple organization to continue to maintain its highly successful status, some still believe that the leadership vacuum left by Jobs took some time to overcome and resulted in a somewhat sluggish transition. And again, the impact of the charismatic leader depends on whether the vision is a positive, affirming one or a negative, dysfunctional one (sometimes masquerading as a positive one). Expanding our pool of identified charismatic leaders, consider that those meeting the definitional criteria of charismatic leadership alongside Gandhi, Mandela, King, and others are Hitler, Jim Jones, and Pol Pot. All were overwhelmingly inspirational, able to launch and sustain incredibly powerful movements supported by loyal, devoted followers. The nature of the visions they put forward and the outcomes they achieved could not be more different.

Transformational leadership is a type of leadership that focuses on the development of relationships with others that elevates them to higher levels of professional and perhaps even moral development, encourages and supports change and adaptability, and can result in enhanced performance and, of course, acceptance of change (Sosik, 2018). This leadership style, so defined, is often considered the most desirable form of leadership, and most good leaders still achieve only some aspects of a true transformational leader. With that said, researchers have identified the "four I's" of transformational leadership as (1) inspirational motivation, (2) idealized influence, (3) intellectual stimulation, and (4) individualized consideration (Avolio & Bass, 2001). "Inspirational motivation" refers to stating and identifying a future desired state or situation – a bold vision of the future – and fully describing a plan to achieve it. "Idealized influence" refers to efforts made to gain the trust, confidence, respect, and devotion from followers while setting and being the example of high standards of professional conduct. "Intellectual stimulation" refers to a leader's questioning current environmental situations (i.e., the status quo) and encouraging continuous and ongoing innovation to ensure improvement. "Individualized consideration" applies to a leader who strongly encourages and assists their followers to achieve their full potential while also mentoring them and appreciating their individuality and their diversity.

In thinking about transformational leadership, and encouraging others to exhibit these behaviors, the expectation may appear daunting. In fact, researchers admit that there may be relatively few individuals who ever fully achieve the idealized definition of true transformational leadership. But being led by someone who is to some extent a transformational leader, or is striving to be such, could enable and support many of the identified individual-level solutions to burnout, while also obviously providing a conduit for both the social support and the systems-level process changes (e.g., adjustments to workload procedures) that help to mitigate burnout.

Some noted examples of individuals identified as transformational leaders throughout history include Queen Elizabeth I of England, Alexander the Great, and, more recently, Nelson Mandela (Johannsen, 2021). There would not be a British Commonwealth without Queen Elizabeth I. Her leadership and willingness to forge alliances was essential to transforming the known world. Alexander, while ruthless in his conquering of nations, certainly did transform people and cultures along the way.

Note that some individuals, like Nelson Mandela, often show up on lists of both transformational and charismatic leaders. When a leader is able to inspire passionate followership and also achieve a major cultural transformation, they fit the criteria of both "forms" of leadership. The two forms are by no means mutually exclusive. One could certainly be charismatic without making major cultural or organizational transformation, but the iconic transformational leaders never acted alone. They inspired enough followers to join them in their vision and then worked with them to realize it.

The third leadership type may be fairly identified at times as weak or even absent leadership. Specifically, laissez-faire leadership is a generally considered a form of non-leadership, or hands-off in the extreme. Laissez-faire leadership is seen in the Michael Scott character of the TV show *The Office*, where the leader takes the lazy approach to leading, and is essentially absent from their duties, if their duties are even defined clearly. Such leaders are leaders in name only.

But, importantly, there is another side to laissez-faire leadership, where a more mature and largely self-managing team experiences an intentionally more hands-off or delegated style of leadership from their leader (Hersey & Blanchard, 1974; Thompson & Vecchio, 2009). Under the circumstances where a leader has a well-established, longer-term team that they have developed to the point that the team no longer needs daily direction or supervision, their job is more about so-called boundary management (i.e., managing relationships between the team and other internal and external groups) and delegating high levels of authority to team members. For example, a physician may have a team of nurses and physician assistants who have worked with the physician, and with each other, for many years. In doing so, over time they can develop a shared mental model of what needs to be done under numerous varying circumstances. In the case of such a mature team, the leader generally does not need to direct behavior, but essentially holds the team to a standard of excellence and delegates tasks as needed. The leader manages from the boundaries of the team, coming in and providing direction only when needed. This is not a laissez-faire, absentee leader. It is a fully appropriate "hands-off" approach to leading a mature team. Note too that if the leader of a more mature, competent team becomes too hands-on and directive, telling team members how to do things that they fully know how to do, the leader can be perceived as a micromanager, which is never a good thing.

Needless to say, most leaders are not 100 percent charismatic, transformational, or laissez-faire. The vast majority of leaders exhibit styles that are somewhere in between or are blends of the three primary styles. They may generally prefer to operate in one of the classic styles, or are more comfortable there, but there are not sharp boundaries between the styles. More specifically, and critically, effective leaders must adapt their style flexibly to the needs of the individual or team they are leading, often engaging in quite different styles as needed (Rahbi et al., 2017). As we will see, teams at different levels of development require quite different styles of leadership. In general, though, in terms of burnout, the research is clear that followers of charismatic leaders and especially transformational leaders generally have lower incidence of burnout than those whose leaders are more laissez-faire (De Hoogh & Den Hartog, 2009; Hildenbrand, Sacramento, & Binnewies, 2018). In other words, if a physician is in a leadership role, they have the opportunity to engage in more of the charismatic and transformational leadership behaviors, thereby helping reduce their followers' burnout.

As an important side note, efforts to lead more effectively also interact with the previous solutions discussed. For example, perhaps most fascinating is the interaction of followers' personality factors with these leadership types (De Hoogh & Den Hartog, 2009). According to the research by De Hoogh and Den Hartog , individuals with lower openness to experience (the openness factor in the predominant Five Factor model of personality) benefit more from transformational leadership exhibited by their leader than those who are higher in openness to experience. This serves as an important reminder that as we move up the levels of intervention from individual to team to system, there are in turn trickle-down effects that will affect the overall incidence of burnout. As we have emphasized, the three levels of intervention strategy are themselves interdependent. A well-led team can promote individual strategies and lobby for system change in order to reduce burnout risk.

Leading and Developing Teams through Their Growth Stages

When well led, teams amplify the effectiveness of their component individuals (Chedrawy, 2020). When poorly led, teams fail to develop and fail to perform, and their overall output and effectiveness may be less than the sum of their component individuals (Stockwell et al., 2005). Indeed, poor teamwork can actually increase stress and introduce errors into a system, other things being equal. Poor teamwork can be a primary source of stress and error, as indicated by our discussion in Chapter 4. Further, a truism in business is "Leadership makes all the difference." It certainly does in the case of teams!

The *Oxford English Dictionary* defines team as "a group of players forming one side in a competitive game or sport." A more comprehensive definition from the *Encyclopedia of Industrial and Organizational Psychology* states that work teams are complex social dynamic entities characterized by having two or more members. Teams hold meaningful goal interdependencies, interact routinely, interact adaptively, and should share a common vision. Teams are often organized hierarchically, usually have a limited life span, and have distributed expertise across the team members. Additionally, they typically engage in cycles of performance and are embedded in an organization that influences their procedures and performance (Salas et al., 2017). Of particular emphasis here is the hierarchical structure present in teams, distinguishing team leader from followers.

For long-term teams – that is, teams that will be a stable working unit over a period of time – the leader has the responsibility of leading the team through predictable stages of development, necessarily drawing on different leader behaviors with intentional flexibility over time. One of the most widely subscribed models was developed by psychologist Bruce Tuckman in the 1960s. According to the classic Tuckman model (Tuckman, 1965), teams go through an initial stage of "forming" in which the leader covers the essential expectations as identified above and ensures that team members have the training and other resources they need to fulfill their individual roles and support each other's efforts toward common goals. Depending on the complexity of the work, and the skill and experience level of the team members at the outset, the forming stage can last for months. The progression through the stages is not a smooth, linear process. In fact, the second stage can look like a step back. As the team starts to work together on common goals, conflicts may appear. As team members work more interdependently with each other, personality differences and associated behavioral differences may surface ("Jack is kind of a know-it-all.... I don't like his arrogant, superior approach.... I have just as much knowledge and experience as he does.... Carla is the weak link on this team ... she is not holding up her end.... Tony is stand-offish and hard to read ... is he "in" or not?"). Additionally, it is common in this second growth stage for team members to develop conflicts with the team leader ("She is not giving us enough direction.... We are not clear on what we are supposed to do or how to do it.... I feel like we are being set up to fail," or, at the other extreme, "She is still over our shoulders telling us what to do.... She is a micro-manager.... Why doesn't she trust us?... I thought we were supposed to be self-directing"). In this second stage, identified appropriately as "storming," the leader must address destructive conflicts and assure the team that they can get through internal strife in service to the overall mission of the team. The leader must understand that the storming stage is a common and natural part of the growth process for teams (sometimes called the "teenage years" of the team) and that it does not represent a failure in team concept. The leader must also not "take it personally" when there is grumbling and dissension in the ranks. It is crucially important that the team be well led during this stage, with clear direction from the leader, but also with more autonomy for the growing team. A failure to lead the team through this turbulent time means no more growth occurs. Once the team is led past the conflict stage, members begin to feel part of something larger than themselves. They begin to establish a sense of identity with the team as well as norms of behavior for themselves and their teammates, identifying "how we will behave and what we expect of each other." This predictable developmental stage is called the "norming" stage and marks a healthy, mature team. In some settings, teams are led to a final stage of self-sufficiency called the "performing" stage where they can function fairly independently of the leader, allowing the leader to operate for the most part in the boundary-manager role that we identified earlier as a positive example of the laissez-faire style. In highly regulated, HRO-type work settings, that ultimate stage of self-direction is generally not a realistic goal. Airline crews don't function independently of a captain; nuclear control room crews are still led by a senior reactor operator; and a surgical team follows the lead of the head surgeon.

In some healthcare settings, such as a nursing home/long-term care facility or a primary care physician's office, long-term, stable care teams can be led and developed gradually to the point of norming, and even performing, in the way indicated above. In many other healthcare settings, however, team composition can frequently shift. A surgical team or an ICU critical care team may have revolving membership, with members rotating in and out frequently. In such familiar situations, the role of the leader becomes especially critical. The leader must establish a norming or performing team in a matter of minutes, not months. How is that accomplished?

When ad hoc, frequently changing, "unstable" (in team membership) teams are the rule, there are two critical requirements for quickly establishing team effectiveness. First, the leader must be totally clear and explicit in establishing and communicating expectations as to how the team will function, who is in what role, how the team will communicate with each other, and so on. Second, clear protocols and procedures must be set that everyone is familiar with beforehand, that is, systems support, which we will address in subsequent chapters. Team members in such short-term teams must bring that knowledge of the guidelines into a new team, and those guidelines must be articulated and amplified by the leader.

As an example, the challenge of the frequently changing team has been prominent in the airlines for many years. As new crews are formed, usually every month, established and endorsed protocols must be set that enable the leader (captain) to form a new operational unit (cockpit crew) very quickly; everyone on the team must know what to expect. This is the same challenge faced by many teams in healthcare. While the ideal is to have a stable, durable team (as with nuclear control-room teams), where that is not possible, the team development process must be radically truncated, by clear direction and understood protocols. There isn't time to "figure it out."

Team Leadership, Leader Member Exchange, and Burnout

Team leadership is all about creating and managing the conditions for team members to work effectively with each other in a collaborative manner. Since the collaborative teamwork environment is the subject of the next chapter, we'll focus here only on one particular leadership theory that provides a starting point for much of the collaboration literature. Specifically, it is important to understand how leader-member exchange theory (LMX) explains how leaders and their followers can assist one another in performing effectively and, as they build their working relationship, in alleviating burnout (Thomas & Lankau, 2009). If a leader demonstrates caring and support, encouragement, clear communication, and so on, we assume that their followers will reciprocate. And that is exactly what leader-member exchange theory is all about. Simply put, LMX states that leaders maintain their hierarchical position in groups through the development and maintenance of relationships with members of their group or team, based on the principle of reciprocity. Their behaviors induce reactions by their followers. Thus, the relationship becomes mutually interdependent and reciprocal (Thomas & Lankau, 2009).

In brief, LMX theory posits that leaders and followers automatically develop relationships as they work together, take some measure of responsibility for one another's actions as they make decisions together, and so on. If these relationships are positive, based in part on ideal leader behavioral strategies such as charismatic or transformational leadership, then the mutually supportive relationships between leader and members have strong potential to augment overall performance while mitigating undesirable outcomes such as stress and burnout (e.g., Lee, 2011). Note that an expectation inherent in LMX theory is that the supportive "exchange" between leader and followers is a model for the same level of reciprocal exchange among the team members themselves. Such a cohesive, collaborative team environment is a known key driver of individual well-being and a strong mitigator of burnout. If we do better in our teams, as leaders and followers, we'll thereby have more resources for our individual-level strategies as well.

Physician Team Leadership and Performance

Key strategies for mitigating burnout at the team level include being a better team leader by employing both charismatic and transformational leadership styles to the extent possible, employing flexible leadership strategies for the development of the team, and recognizing the leader-member exchange relationships that naturally emerge and can be a tremendous source of social support. Research on the effects of leadership training on physicians in academic medical centers (Straus et al., 2013) has shown that the availability of such targeted, high-quality leadership training correlated with the academic rank, hospital leadership position, and publication success of physicians who received such training. Additionally, these findings of the benefits of leadership training for physicians are also confirmed in similar studies with other healthcare workers, such as nurses (Cummings et al., 2018).

Summing Up

In sum, leadership matters! And people vary greatly in the way they lead. Some may lean strongly and consistently toward one or another style. Others may be more flexible in adapting their style to the circumstances. However, we know that transformational leaders are able to lead in such a way as to reduce the burnout of their people. This is true throughout history, in recent research, and likely in any given healthcare environment. Additionally, we know that an exchange relationship between a leader and a follower helps enable the social support processes we've talked about in previous chapters. Thus, leader-member exchange is an important method for enabling better coping with stress and thus for reducing burnout in teams and the individuals who work in them.

The COVID-19 Effect

COVID-19 has strongly demonstrated the importance of leadership in crisis situations. As mentioned in relation to HROs, leadership has the potential to adapt and enable team performance to avoid the negative outcomes that should not occur, but sometimes do. In reviewing experiences that healthcare leaders have had in managing the COVID-19 crisis, several leadership behaviors emerged as especially important. These crucial leader behaviors prominently include planning and coordination, team situational monitoring, communication (always!), and adaptation to the ever-changing landscape of the virus (Nicola et al., 2020). For example, even as the Delta variant of the coronavirus began to rise and create problems for residents of southwest Missouri, healthcare leaders and their teams adapted, appropriately transferring patients to other locations, adapting to rapidly changing situations on the ground, and in general enabling care in ways not needed previous to the crisis (Holman, 2021). These examples demonstrate in specific terms the value of positive leadership in crisis situations such as the pandemic and how such leadership can enable better patient care, while monitoring the well-being of the care providers.

Key Takeaways

- Leadership is essential to mitigating and stemming the tide of burnout in our physicians and their healthcare teams
- Leadership styles vary and according to classic typologies include charismatic, transformational, and laissez-faire approaches
- Most leaders prefer some styles over others, but must adapt their style to fit the needs of their teams, including the need to reduce burnout.
- Leader-member exchange is all about building relationships between leaders and followers, which can increase social support and thereby help to reduce burnout

REFERENCES

Avolio, B. J., & Bass, B. M. (eds.). (2001). *Developing Potential across a Full Range of Leadership: Cases on Transactional and Transformational Leadership.* Mahwah, NJ: Psychology Press.

Chedrawy, E., (2020). Well-led teams: The big payoff. *Physician Leadership Journal, 7*(6), 12.

Cummings, G. G., Tate, K., Lee, S., Wong, C. A., Paananen, T., Micaroni, S. P., & Chatterjee, G. E. (2018). Leadership styles and outcome patterns for the nursing workforce and work environment: A systematic review. *International Journal of Nursing Studies, 85*, 19–60.

De Hoogh, A. H., & Den Hartog, D. N. (2009). Neuroticism and locus of control as moderators of the relationships of charismatic and autocratic leadership with burnout. *Journal of Applied Psychology, 94*(4), 1058.

Gentry, W. A. (2016). *Be the Boss Everyone Wants to Work For: A Guide for New Leaders.* Oakland, CA: Berrett-Koehler Publishers.

Hersey, P., & Blanchard, K. H. (1974). So you want to know your leadership style? *Training & Development Journal, 28*(2), 22–37.

Hildenbrand, K., Sacramento, C. A., & Binnewies, C. (2018). Transformational leadership and burnout: The role of thriving and followers' openness to experience. *Journal of Occupational Health Psychology, 23*(1), 31.

Holman, G. J. (2021, June 30). Health care "breaking point": Cox confirms some Springfield COVID-19 patients transferred to St. Louis, Kansas City. *Springfield News-Leader.* www.news-leader.com/story/news/local/ozarks/2021/06/29/springfield-covid-delta-variant-missouri-hospitals-cox-some-patients-transferred-vaccines/7787970002/.

House, R. J. (1976). A 1976 theory of charismatic leadership. Working Paper Series 76-06.

Janse, B. (2019). Leader-Member Exchange Theory (LMX). Toolshero. www.toolshero.com/management/leader-member-exchange-theory-lmx/#:~:text=The%20Leader%2DMember%20Exchange%20Theory%20(LMX)%2C%20also%20called,to%20growth%20or%20hinder%20development.

Johannsen, M. (2021, May 23). 125 Transformational leaders: Lists of famous ones from many countries. Legacee. www.legacee.com/transformational_leadership/list-of-leaders#4-three-great-transformational-leaders.

Judge, T. A., Fluegge Woolf, E., Hurst, C., & Livingston, B. (2006). Charismatic and transformational leadership: A review and an agenda for future research. *Zeitschrift für Arbeits-und Organisationspsychologie A&O, 50*(4), 203–214.

Lee, K. E. (2011). Moderating effects of leader-member exchange (LMX) on job burnout in dietitians and chefs of institutional foodservice. *Nutrition Research and Practice, 5*(1), 80–87.

McManus, M. R. (2021). 10 far-out charismatic leaders (and the trouble they caused). HowStuffWorks. https://people.howstuffworks.com/10-charismatic-leaders.htm#:~:text=What%20are%20some%20examples%20of,all%20examples%20of%20charismatic%20leaders.

Nicola, M., Sohrabi, C., Mathew, G., Kerwan, A., Al-Jabir, A., Griffin, M., Agha, M., & Agha, R. (2020). Health policy and leadership models during the COVID-19 pandemic: A review. *International Journal of Surger, 81*, 122–129. https://doi.org/10.1016/j.ijsu.2020.07.026.

Nguyen, S. (2017, December 10). The dangers of charismatic leaders. Workplace Psychology. https://workplacepsychology.net/2010/11/26/the-dangers-of-charismatic-leaders/.

Rahbi, D. A., Khalid, K., & Khan, M. (2017). The effects of leadership styles on team motivation. *Academy of Strategic Management Journal, 16*(3).

Salas, E., Reyes, D. L., & Woods, A. L. (2017). The assessment of team performance: Observations and needs. In *Innovative Assessment of Collaboration*, ed. A. A. Von Davier, M. Zhu, & P. C. Kyllonen (pp. 21–36). Cham: Springer.

Sosik, J. J., Arenas, F. J., Chun, J. U., & Ete, Z. (2018). Character into action: How officers demonstrate strengths with transformational leadership. *Air & Space Power Journal, 32*(3), 4–26.

Stockwell, D. C., Pollack, M. M., Turenne, W. M., Gibson, C. L., & Slonim, A. D. (2005). Physician team leadership affects clinical achievement in the intensive care unit (ICU). *Critical Care Medicine, 33*(12), A2.

Straus, S. E., Soobiah, C., & Levinson, W. (2013). The impact of leadership training programs on physicians in academic medical centers: A systematic review. *Academic Medicine, 88*(5), 710–723.

Thomas, C. H., & Lankau, M. J. (2009). Preventing burnout: The effects of LMX and mentoring on socialization, role stress, and burnout. *Human Resource Management, 48*(3), 417–432.

Thompson, G., & Vecchio, R. P. (2009). Situational leadership theory: A test of three versions. *The Leadership Quarterly, 20*(5), 837–848.

Tuckman, B. W. (1965). Development sequence in small groups. *Psychological Bulletin, 63*(6), 384–399.

Weber, M. (1947). *The Theory of Social and Economic Organization*. New York: Simon and Schuster.

Yukl, G. (2010). *Leadership in Organizations*, 7th ed. Upper Saddle River, NJ: Prentice Hall.

CHAPTER 10

Solution #6: Ensure Collaborating Team Members

You know, I really couldn't be good at caring for my patients if I couldn't rely on my fellow physicians.

—Occupational medicine physician

As made clear in the previous chapter on Solution #5, the team leader is the single most responsible party in developing and managing a team. Leadership always makes the difference (Avolio & Bass, 2001). But the team leader certainly can't do it alone. The leader can (and must) set the expectations and guidelines for the team, whether the team is long-term or ad hoc, but team members themselves are obviously critical partners in this process. They must understand how to function interdependently and fully embrace their role as productive and supportive team members. Indeed, the supportive attitudes and behaviors of team members are essential for the enactment of the leader's vision, which must be a shared vision for the team, as we will address later. Whatever their specialty, whatever contributing role they play on the team, team members must understand how their work impacts and is impacted by the work of the others on the team, how they are interrelated. They are not just an individual contributor; as they go about their assigned tasks they are also a helper and supporter of others. They work interdependently. They collaborate. Teamwork and collaboration are key for each team member and for the success of the team overall. To our main point here, teamwork and collaboration are essential for optimum performance and also assist with the mitigation of burnout among team members and their leader.

What Are Teamwork and Collaboration in General?

Teamwork has been defined variously by many different researchers in the social sciences over the years. Some define teamwork simply as the enactment of teamwork processes intended to support overall effective team

132

performance (Driskell et al., 2018). More specifically, teamwork can be defined as "the integration of individuals' efforts toward the accomplishment of a shared goal" (Mathieu, Maynard, Rapp, & Gilson, 2008; p. 458). Many researchers and team scholars view teamwork within the general framework of an input-process-output (IPO) model of team effectiveness (Mathieu et al., 2008). An IPO model postulates that inputs (e.g., team member characteristics, team-level factors, and contextual factors) have an influence on team output (i.e., team effectiveness by a variety of measures). However, this input-output relationship is mediated by the processes that take place within team interaction. A luminary in the groups and teams literature, Richard Hackman (2012), stated that "the core idea of the model is that input states affect group outcomes via the interaction that takes place among members" (p. 431). In other words, internal team processes (teamwork) are the means through which team resources are directed to achieve desired team outcomes. In the case of healthcare, team outputs would include the quality and overall effectiveness of patient care (e.g., no errors), ultimate patient satisfaction, the commitment of the team to achieving team goals, and, critically, their commitment to each other.

Given the importance of team processes, it may come as no surprise that one of the most thoroughly studied team processes, and among the most critical, is collaboration. While the distinction may appear to be a subtle one, collaboration is commonly identified as a component, element, or subtype of teamwork in which team members coordinate their activities directly among themselves, without requiring the close direction or supervision of their leader. It is essentially peer-to-peer teamwork, typical of a mature (norming or performing) team. It should be noted that the terms "collaboration" and "coordination" are often used interchangeably in the research literature on the science of teams. We use the term "collaboration" here, but will reference works by those who use the term "coordination" as well. Collaboration occurs when two or more team members engage in a joint activity to achieve a shared goal (Bedwell et al., 2012), sometimes in the "process of orchestrating the sequence and timing of independent actions" (Marks et al., 2001, pp. 367–368). In order to effectively collaborate as a team, team leaders and especially team members need to attend to matching team member resources to task requirements, regulate the pace of team activities, and coordinate the response and sequencing of team member activities (Driskell et al., 2018).

While the leader is the primary manager of the processes of teamwork, each team member must be comfortable in proactively providing some measure of collaboration as well. Communication is always central, as team members must speak up and keep each other informed of current status, changes, and potential or actual problems. Effective communication behaviors include exchanging information in a timely manner, acknowledgment of information received, double-checking that the intent of messages was received and understood, clarifying ambiguity, and the appropriate use of verbal and nonverbal cues (Salas et al., 2009). In a meta-analysis of information sharing and team performance, Mesmer-Magnus and DeChurch (2009) found overall that information sharing was positively related to team performance and that sharing uniquely held information was more predictive of team performance than simply sharing a greater amount of information. Thus, team members must ask questions as needed, not only of each other but of their leader as well. They must also be willing to volunteer information, as needed. In order for team members to communicate effectively, as identified in the research literature, the team leader must set the expectation that all can speak up, and must allow and encourage team-member input. Unless the leader explicitly sets such ground rules for the team, members are less likely to "take the chance" to speak up. And if the leader has set the expectation of open information-sharing, it is crucially important that when a team member does speak up, even if questioning the leader, that team member is rewarded (and not punished!) for speaking up. Furthermore, through the implementation of strategies of open communication, team members must ensure that they and their teammates are all working "on the same page" with the same shared mental model from the information exchanged throughout the collaborative process.

Teamwork and Collaboration in Healthcare Teams

In recent years, there has been a huge surge of interest in applying general principles of teamwork and the specific teamwork process of collaboration into the arena of healthcare, our focus throughout this book. For example, at this time, a quick Google search found 38 million hits for the combined key terms of teamwork and healthcare, with 4.7 million from just one year (2020). At the turn of the twenty-first century, there were only 4,700 hits on the topic, suggesting that a major boom in interest has occurred. One reason for this boom is the increasing visibility of the medical error problem as previously discussed, and the knowledge that the well-led, smoothly functioning team has great potential to reduce error. Perhaps as no surprise, when it was estimated that 44,000 Americans die each year as a result of medical errors, the landmark Institute of Medicine (2000) report, *To Err Is Human*, called for improved teamwork as an essential strategy to reduce errors in health care. This call was embraced, and in 2016 Hughes and colleagues found that team training interventions were effective at multiple levels of analysis, including individual (e.g., individual learning), team (e.g., teamwork performance), and organizational (e.g., safety climate) levels. As a more specific example, when Weaver and colleagues (2010) provided a training to improve teamwork in operating room teams they observed significant improvement in the quality of briefings and the frequency of specific effective teamwork behaviors during actual cases.

Let's now turn our attention to several further benefits of teamwork and collaboration in healthcare, before providing key suggestions as to what physicians and other healthcare providers can do to improve teamwork and collaboration, including the closely related mitigation of burnout and reduction of errors.

Further Benefits of Teamwork in Healthcare

Starting with the broader domain of overall teamwork in healthcare, research has identified two major areas that experience especially dramatic benefits as a result of effective teamwork: patient care outcomes and healthcare worker outcomes. In terms of patient care, Rosen and colleagues (2018) cite a dramatic increase in the amount of work directly with patients (i.e., increasing patient counts) and find links between the quality of teamwork and the quality and safety of healthcare delivery to patients. Work on patient care outcomes focuses on three primary areas: (1) patient experience (e.g., patient satisfaction), (2) clinical patient outcomes, and (3) the quality (i.e., degree to which treatment plans are consistent with current guidelines, professional etiquette, and the latest professional knowledge) and safety (i.e., reduction of the risk of patient harm that is preventable) of care.

First, patients indicate they have greater positive experiences with their care when the quality of the teamwork is high, particularly for inpatient facilities (Lyu, Wick, Housman, Freischlag, & Makary, 2013). While there may be many underlying reasons, the bottom line is that better teamwork is consistently associated with better ratings by patients.

Second, perhaps of most interest to physicians considering the effects of teamwork on care plans, there are numerous studies showing that teamwork is associated with positive effects on clinical outcomes for patients. For example, Gittell and colleagues found that patients receiving care from teams with higher levels of mutual trust, clearly defined roles, and effective information exchange procedures also experienced increased postoperative functioning, shorter stays in clinical in-patient settings, and lower levels of postoperative pain (Gittell et al., 2000). Given the ongoing opioid crisis, the latter may serve as reason enough on its own to embrace strategies for developing more effective teamwork among healthcare providers. Looking at comparable studies outside the United States, Lyubovnikova and colleagues (2015) performed a large-scale survey with the UK National Health Service. They found that healthcare workers who reported conducting their work in effective teams also reported lower rates of errors and lower patient mortality overall.

Third, in terms of both quality and safety of care, a variety of studies confirm the critically important nature of team communication in reducing risks. Patients receiving care from teams with poor communication are almost five times as likely, according to a study by Mazzocco and colleagues (2009), to experience complications or even death during an in-patient hospital visit. Further, one observational study of surgical teams found that 30 percent of team interactions included some failure in communication, a communication breakdown of some type (Lingard et al., 2004). As a side note on this point, John has had the opportunity to fly in the jump seat in the cockpit on numerous flights with major domestic airlines, in order to observe and assess team processes, including communication, in action. In most cases, there was at least one minor miscommunication, and sometimes several. In all of those cases, using the specific techniques of effective teamwork that they had been trained in, members of the team quickly identified and corrected the minor miscues. Such is the power of effective teams; properly trained members quickly identify and correct such errors and quickly get the team back on the same page, without consequence.

Although a failure in communication in the healthcare setting may be as simple as the nonthreatening issue of the location of the waste disposal bin for biowaste, it could also be a failure to communicate an essential step in the surgical procedure resulting in a hospital-acquired condition or worse. Thus, teamwork in healthcare settings from that of the physician to the phlebotomist or any other team members is truly critically important for the care of patients. Interestingly, the benefits do not stop here.

In terms of physician and healthcare worker outcomes, teamwork also creates a more positive, engaging, and resilient work environment. The evidence suggests that hospitals in which staff report higher levels of teamwork, with effective leaders who define and communicate clear roles and expectations, have lower rates of workplace injuries and illness, see fewer experiences of workplace harassment and violence, and overall lower levels of staff intent to leave the organization (Lyubovnikova et al., 2015). As we will discuss in the next chapter, the teamwork climate of a work unit is highly related to the level of engagement that staff feel in their work, such that units with a strongly positive teamwork climate also have staff with a strong commitment to, and sense of ownership of, their job responsibilities (Biddison, Paine, Murakami, Herzke, & Weaver, 2016).

Perhaps most important for the reader of this book, teamwork quality is inversely related to the level of burnout experienced by physicians and staff members (Bowers, Nijman, Simpson, & Jones, 2011). That is, units with poor teamwork tend to have physicians and staff with higher reported levels of physical, mental, and emotional fatigue – burnout. Further, for teams in the United Kingdom, better teamwork, including greater role clarity among multidisciplinary teams, is associated with higher job satisfaction (Carpenter, Schneider, Brandon, & Wooff, 2003). Thus, teamwork makes for healthier and happier physicians, who experience lower burnout overall. But what specific processes within overall teamwork are driving those positive outcomes? The main answer is collaboration.

The Critical Role of Collaboration in Healthcare Teams

Collaboration in the healthcare literature actually encompasses more processes than mentioned so far in relation to communication and coordination of tasks among team members. According to a review of literature by Morley and colleagues (2017), collaboration within teams includes the following for elements in healthcare settings:

1. Coordination in working to achieve shared goals
2. Cooperation in contributing to the team, while understanding and valuing the contributions of all team members
3. Shared decision-making that relies on negotiation, communication, openness, trust, and respectful power balance
4. Partnerships that include open and respectful relationships cultivated over time where team members work equitably together

When these elements come together in a meaningful way, the benefits include improvements in quality of care, patient engagement, patient safety, and health and well-being of physicians, staff, and the organization. Further, as these elements are introduced or enhanced in a team-based environment, they should augment the teamwork that is already occurring. Thus, teamwork and collaboration go hand in hand.

In terms of quality of care, there is both qualitative and quantitative support for improving the peer-to-peer collaboration within the team. First, qualitatively speaking, collaborative teams demonstrate improved sharing of evidence-based practice across professions, make better decisions, and are more likely to engage in creative and innovative strategies for care (Pike et al., 1993). Second, quantitatively speaking, the evidence suggests that collaborative teamwork is consistently associated with reduced length of hospital stay, greater compliance with standards for prescribing drugs, better audit results, and improved symptom and psychosocial management (Elsayem et al., 2004; Reeves et al., 2011). Essentially, healthcare experts across a number of professions conclude that collaboratively practicing teams are more responsive, efficient, and considerate of patients and their families, and care improves (Schmitt et al., 2011).

Summing Up

Based on the definitions and practices of teamwork and collaboration presented throughout the chapter so far, we provide here in summary form some best practices for mitigating burnout through the use of effective teams. Through the many decades of research and applied work on teams, including work with surgical teams, physician groups, and nursing teams, seven teamwork and collaboration practices can be recommended by us and also by team researchers, along with examples of what they might look like in a physician and healthcare setting.

1. *Effective teams adopt a shared leadership model that establishes a climate of ongoing, open, and transparent communication.* The previous chapter explored the various leadership styles and behaviors that make a leader effective and have the ability to reduce burnout among team members. However, the most effective teams are led to the point that they actually adopt a shared leadership model where all those behaviors suggested in Chapter 9 are, at times, enacted by each and every team member. Each team member can and should serve as the leader when conditions arise for them to do so, and doing so can foster the environment that is essential for effective team collaboration, thereby reducing burnout (Lovelace, Manz, & Alves, 2007).

Again, communication is key in both teamwork and collaboration within teams. Team leaders and particularly influential team members need to recognize that their leadership in the team can make it hard for others to speak up, ask questions, challenge a direction, or otherwise dissent (Rosen et al., 2018). Therefore, team leaders and members who share some of the leadership responsibilities for the team must establish and honor guidelines that make it acceptable for members of the team to speak up. Doing so will help to establish a more psychologically safe team environment that is essential for true collaboration to occur. Thus, the leaders guarantee "psychological safety," which is crucial for team effectiveness. Under the shared leadership paradigm, all team members need to be able to speak up, professionally and respectfully, without fear of repercussions. In other words, as an effective communication strategy and safe communication environment are coestablished between the team leader and members, the research and our experience tell us that holding back information will cease to occur, discussions will begin to occur more openly and honestly, and the critical teamwork process of true collaboration will flourish.

In a healthcare setting, such a communication environment would mean, among other things, that physicians and nurses would be more open and transparent in sharing patient information. For example, if new developments occurred over the course of the day, and the on-call physician is called in, new information should be shared with them verbally from the on-duty nurse or others in the care team. Reliance on electronic records to be both up-to-date and comprehensive is problematic, and an effective team communication climate ensures an additional and, we think, more effective information exchange pathway.

2. Team members themselves give and seek feedback. Team members should use agreed-on communication strategies and even specific agreed-on language for feedback. For example, in nuclear operations, a supervisor/ senior operator will give a direction to a control operator by first calling that individual's name (getting attention), giving the direction (clearly), and then requiring a specific "repeat back" (to ensure that the direction was received and is being followed). Other HROs require similar check-and-verify feedback strategies. It is not acceptable for a team leader to call out a direction, get no response, and assume that the direction was clear, heard, and acted on. Implementing such a strategy within a team of physicians and nurses would ensure that in a high-stakes situation with a patient, errors are eliminated because the confirmation process would ensure both a timely catching of and a timely correction of the error.

3. Team members continually watch out for each other. While each team member has specific roles and assignments, they all help to ensure that others are enacting their roles according to plan. Each is accountable not only for their individual role, but to some extent for the roles that other members of the team are playing. They know what to expect of each other, and they audit not only their own performance but the performance of their teammates. As an example, in nuclear operations some teams have identified what they call "three-step syndrome," in which a team member is moving around the control room and appears to be "busy" but is "three steps behind" where the team is. Operators are trained to watch out for such examples of team dysfunction and correct them when they occur.

4. *Team members operate with shared mental models, or "big picture" awareness to ensure that everyone is on the same page.* Mental models are individually held understandings about the current situation that, when shared, form a common understanding, a common database that helps team members function collaboratively in their work environments (Fiore et al., 2013). Stable teams that have worked together well, communicated effectively, and built over time shared mental models are positioned to work seamlessly through virtually any situation or emergency. When the situation at hand is novel and unfamiliar, it becomes critical for team members to communicate their individual models, their individual situational awareness, and come to a common understanding, a shared mental model of the situation they are in, and of what actions they should take. As we noted earlier, in nuclear operations, whether in the simulator or in the actual control room, when a team is dealing with an off-normal condition, any member of the team can call out "update," with a raised hand, and the team comes together in the middle of the control room to ensure that everyone knows the game plan. All know what each one knows. There is an agreed-on, accurate shared mental model.

In addition to a shared mental model of the situation a team is in, an additional shared mental model that is particularly important for physician healthcare teams is a shared understanding of who on the interdisciplinary team knows what. That is, who has what expertise and who must be consulted as the team works collaboratively to address a patient's needs. The areas of expertise within a healthcare team are often defined by roles, but long-term teams whose members know each other well also recognize expertise, in whatever form it might take, as an essential input to the team.

6. *Team members take responsibility for outcomes of the whole team, not just for their individual contributing part.* Teams exist to achieve common goals. It is the "whole," the successful accomplishment of the team's assignment, the outcome that matters. As a cohesive unit, the outcomes are a function of all members working together. Thus, win or lose, make

the last shot or miss, save the patient or not, the buck stops with the collective team.

7. *Team members share the burden of being aware of each other's stress level.* All team members recognize certain times and certain situations in which they are under additional pressure. They are especially focused on watching out for themselves and each other for safe, error-free operation during these peak times. It is important for team members to be mindful of, empathize with, and care for their team members, enough to see when they are stressed or burned out, and be a source of support. For pilots, it is takeoffs and landings. For nuclear control room operators, it is an off-normal situation that might require a shutdown of the reactor. For healthcare providers, it is any intense situation in which quick action must be taken (without all the information needed) and a patient's life may be in the balance.

The COVID-19 Effect

As COVID-19 put dramatic pressure on physicians and healthcare workers at every level, a surprising positive outcome has been observed, namely, increased collaboration (Roth, 2020). In interviewing leaders in healthcare systems across the United States, Roth (2020) found that several things changed that allowed for more collaboration than ever before. Responding to COVID-19 required unprecedented innovation, flexibility, and speed. Thus, discipline-specific silos that often exist between hospital departments came down. There was a sudden need to shift strategies (e.g., the sudden surge in telehealth) and to share resources that required health systems to coordinate and, in some cases, operate as a single entity, rather than as separate hospitals stockpiling supplies. Deep collaborations were forged in the fires of necessity.

Key Takeaways

- Teamwork and collaboration are distinct processes that are essential to the success of physicians and other healthcare workers as they care for patients and each other.
- When teamwork and collaboration occur, patients have better experiences, and those who care for them, prominently including their physicians, also experience better health outcomes.
- There are meaningful, actionable steps to improving both teamwork and collaboration among healthcare providers, including providing

feedback, watching out for one another, and taking responsibility for individual and team actions. Such steps can ultimately result in a powerful, positive culture of teamwork.

• Teamwork and collaboration have flourished during the crisis of COVID-19, as necessity required unprecedentedly quick innovation, flexibility, and sharing of resources.

REFERENCES

Avolio, B. J., & Bass, B. M. (eds.). (2001). *Developing Potential across a Full Range of Leadership: Cases on Transactional and Transformational Leadership.* Mahwah, NJ: Psychology Press.

Bedwell, W. L., Wildman, J. L., DiazGranados, D., Salazar, M., Kramer, W. S., & Salas, E. (2012). Collaboration at work: An integrative multilevel conceptualization. *Human Resource Management Review, 22*(2), 128–145.

Biddison, E. L. D., Paine, L., Murakami, P., Herzke, C., & Weaver, S. J. (2016). Associations between safety culture and employee engagement over time: A retrospective analysis. *BMJ Quality & Safety, 25*(1), 31–37.

Bowers, L., Nijman, H., Simpson, A., & Jones, J. (2011). The relationship between leadership, teamworking, structure, burnout and attitude to patients on acute psychiatric wards. *Social Psychiatry and Psychiatric Epidemiology, 46*(2), 143–148. https://doi.org/10.1007/s00127-010-0180-8.

Carpenter, J., Schneider, J., Brandon, T., & Wooff, D. (2003). Working in multidisciplinary community mental health teams: The impact on social workers and health professionals of integrated mental health care. *British Journal of Social Work, 33*(8), 1081–1103.

Carson, J. B., Tesluk, P. E., & Marrone, J. A. (2007). Shared leadership in teams: An investigation of antecedent conditions and performance. *Academy of Management Journal, 50*(5), 1217–1234.

Driskell, J. E., Salas, E., & Driskell, T. (2018). Foundations of teamwork and collaboration. *The American Psychologist, 73*(4), 334–348. https://doi.org/10.1037/amp0000241.

Elsayem, A., Swint, K., Fisch, M. J., Palmer, J. L., Reddy, S., Walker, P., Zhukovsky, D., Knight, P., & Bruera, E. (2004). Palliative care inpatient service in a comprehensive cancer center: Clinical and financial outcomes. *Journal of Clinical Oncology, 22*(10), 2008–2014. https://doi.org/10.1200/JCO.2004.11.003.

Fiore, S. M., Salas, E., & Cannon-Bowers, J. A. (2013). Group dynamics and shared mental model development. In *How People Evaluate Others in Organizations*, ed. M. London (pp. 335–362). Mahwah, NJ: Psychology Press.

Gittell, J. H., Fairfield, K. M., Bierbaum, B., Head, W., Jackson, R., Kelly, M., Laskin, R., Lipson, S., Siliski, J., Thornhill, T., & Zuckerman, J. (2000).

Impact of relational coordination on quality of care, postoperative pain and functioning, and length of stay: A nine-hospital study of surgical patients. *Medical Care, 38*(8), 807–819. https://doi.org/10.1097/00005650-200008000-00005.

Hackman, J. R. (2012). From causes to conditions in group research. *Journal of Organizational Behavior, 33*(3), 428–444.

Hughes, A. M., Gregory, M. E., Joseph, D. L., Sonesh, S. C., Marlow, S. L., Lacerenza, C. N., Benishek, L. E., King, H. B., & Salas, E. (2016). Saving lives: A meta-analysis of team training in healthcare. *The Journal of Applied Psychology, 101*(9), 1266–1304. https://doi.org/10.1037/apl0000120.

Institute of Medicine Committee on Quality of Health Care in America, Kohn, L. T., Corrigan, J. M., & Donaldson, M. S. (eds.). (2000). *To Err Is Human: Building a Safer Health System*. Washington, DC: National Academies Press.

Lingard, L., Espin, S., Whyte, S., Regehr, G., Baker, G. R., Reznick, R., Bohnen, J., Orser, B., Doran, D., & Grober, E. (2004). Communication failures in the operating room: An observational classification of recurrent types and effects. *Quality & Safety in Health Care, 13*(5), 330–334. https://doi.org/10.1136/qhc.13.5.330.

Lovelace, K. J., Manz, C. C., & Alves, J. C. (2007). Work stress and leadership development: The role of self-leadership, shared leadership, physical fitness and flow in managing demands and increasing job control. *Human Resource Management Review, 17*(4), 374–387.

Lyu, H., Wick, E. C., Housman, M., Freischlag, J. A., & Makary, M. A. (2013). Patient satisfaction as a possible indicator of quality surgical care. *JAMA Surgery, 148*(4), 362–367. https://doi.org/10.1001/2013.jamasurg.270.

Lyubovnikova, J., West, M. A., Dawson, J. F., & Carter, M. R. (2015). 24-karat or fool's gold? Consequences of real team and co-acting group membership in healthcare organizations. *European Journal of Work and Organizational Psychology, 24*(6), 929–950.

Marks, M. A., Mathieu, J. E., & Zaccaro, S. J. (2001). A temporally based framework and taxonomy of team processes. *Academy of Management Review, 26*(3), 356–376.

Mathieu, J., Maynard, M. T., Rapp, T., & Gilson, L. (2008). Team effectiveness 1997–2007: A review of recent advancements and a glimpse into the future. *Journal of management, 34*(3), 410–476.

Mazzocco, K., Petitti, D. B., Fong, K. T., Bonacum, D., Brookey, J., Graham, S., Lasky, R. E., Sexton, J. B., & Thomas, E. J. (2009). Surgical team behaviors and patient outcomes. *American Journal of Surgery, 197*(5), 678–685. https://doi.org/10.1016/j.amjsurg.2008.03.002.

Mesmer-Magnus, J. R., & DeChurch, L. A. (2009). Information sharing and team performance: A meta-analysis. *Journal of Applied Psychology, 94*(2), 535.

Morley, L., & Cashell, A. (2017). Collaboration in health care. *Journal of Medical Imaging and Radiation Sciences, 48*(2), 207–216.

Pike, A. W., McHugh, M., Canney, K. C., Miller, N. E., Reiley, P., & Seibert, C. P. (1993). A new architecture for quality assurance: Nurse-physician

collaboration. *Journal of Nursing Care Quality, 7*(3), 1–8. https://doi.org/10
.1097/00001786-199304000-00007.

Reeves, S., Lewin, S., Espin, S., & Zwarenstein, M. (2011). *Interprofessional
Teamwork for Health and Social Care*, vol. 8. Hoboken, NJ: John Wiley &
Sons.

Rosen, M. A., DiazGranados, D., Dietz, A. S., Benishek, L. E., Thompson, D.,
Pronovost, P. J., & Weaver, S. J. (2018). Teamwork in healthcare: Key
discoveries enabling safer, high-quality care. *The American Psychologist, 73*(4),
433–450. https://doi.org/10.1037/amp0000298.

Roth, M. (2020, October 12). The unexpected side effect of COVID-19:
Collaboration. Health Leaders. www.healthleadersmedia.com/innovation/
unexpected-side-effect-covid-19-collaboration.

Salas, E., Almeida, S. A., Salisbury, M., King, H., Lazzara, E. H., Lyons, R.,
Wilson, K. A., Almeida, P. A., & McQuillan, R. (2009). What are the
critical success factors for team training in health care? *Joint Commission
Journal on Quality and Patient Safety, 35*(8), 398–405. https://doi.org/10
.1016/s1553-7250(09)35056-4.

Schmitt, M., Blue, A., Aschenbrener, C. A., & Viggiano, T. R. (2011). Core
competencies for interprofessional collaborative practice: Reforming health
care by transforming health professionals' education. *Academic Medicine, 86*
(11), 1351–1359.

Weaver, S. J., Rosen, M. A., DiazGranados, D., Lazzara, E. H., Lyons, R., Salas,
E., Knych, S. A., McKeever, M., Adler, L., Barker, M., & King, H. B.
(2010). Does teamwork improve performance in the operating room?
A multilevel evaluation. *Joint Commission Journal on Quality and Patient
Safety, 36*(3), 133–142. https://doi.org/10.1016/s1553-7250(10)36022-3.

Solution #7: Establish and Sustain a Positive Team Culture

Pre-pandemic, we used to take lunch breaks together as a team. Well, not all at once, but in shifts. It was kind of the highlight of my day. So much has changed.

—Medical resident

The previous two chapters discussed teamwork-based solutions to the risk of burnout, at the levels of team leadership and team-member teamwork/ collaboration, respectively. Not surprisingly, those two chapters identified many of the key transactional strategies that result in ultimately establishing and sustaining a positive team culture. Remember, teams exist to achieve common goals through their effective leadership and collaborative performance. But there is a crucial social aspect beyond this technical, performance/outcomes aspect of teams. If the team is well led and the team members embrace and act on their role as partners in a collaborative effort, the team can establish a culture not only of performance excellence but also of positivity, mutual respect, and genuine caring for each other. This positive team culture, once established, functions in and of itself as a stress buffer. Even when the work is challenging and high-stakes, as in all HROs, teams that have a positive culture, teams that win, teams that people want to be part of, can be major sources of stress reduction for all members. In this chapter we explore what a positive team culture is, what it looks like generally, and how leadership, collaboration, and other behaviors help establish and sustain the positive team culture. We then explore ways in which physicians can foster a positive team culture for the great benefit of themselves and others on their team.

We briefly discussed earlier the issue of long-term, stable teams versus ad hoc, temporary teams. Many of the ideas and science-based solutions proposed here will speak most directly to teams that are stable and long-term. For example, a primary care physician with their group of physician assistants, nurses, lab techs, administrative personnel, and possibly others would represent a generally stable team. From time to time, of course, people will come and go due to natural attrition and turnover (e.g., found a job elsewhere, retired, or moved to be closer to family). However, in these relatively stable teams, learning each person's personality, what motivates and encourages them, and how to develop them throughout their time with the team is essential and meaningful.

In contrast, within many healthcare settings for a variety of extremely important processes and procedures, ad hoc teams are much more commonly used. In ad hoc teams the composition of the team changes over time and from event to event, sometimes very rapidly. Consider surgical teams and emergency room teams. They are often mixed and matched based on shift changes, vacations, the needs of the patient being worked on, who's available at the moment, lunch schedule, and turnover. In other words, from one day to the next, a physician may be working with many different people, and the makeup of the team, the team dynamics, and the personalities are not the same. Sure, over time, if the pool of personnel overall is stable and small, people will get to know each other and some of the ambiguity and challenge of the ad hoc team environment will subside. But establishing a positive culture will always be more challenging in an ad hoc team environment. Yet it is no less important or rewarding.

What Is a Positive Team Culture?

In order to understand what constitutes a positive team culture, we begin by defining and explaining the concept of organizational culture more broadly. Organizational culture can be defined as the shared set of values, beliefs, and attitudes that guide an organization, represented by the visible artifacts, policies and procedures, mission statements, and other characteristics of the organization, its leadership, and the people therein (Shin et al., 2016). In other words, it's "how we do things around here." We see outward signs of organizational cultures all around us, when we see the golden arches of McDonald's or when we see the big red truck with Coca-Cola written on the side. These symbols (visible artifacts) resonate with the employees who work in the organization, as well as with the general public. Also, each organization has its own rules, policies, procedures, and practices that define how people are expected to work within these companies, including such things as dress codes and promotion procedures, among many other norms. Those physicians who have worked in different medical systems or hospital environments recognize that the experience does indeed differ substantially among these organizations, and a large part of that is driven by the organizational culture, whether it is more open and positive or more closed, and potentially negative or even hostile. We will discuss overall organizational culture a bit more later as we discuss organization and system-level solutions to the burnout problem. For now our focus is a positive *team* culture.

Team culture has been defined as the shared set of values, beliefs, and attitudes that guide team behavior and performance (Willard-Grace et al., 2014). The team culture comprises norms that determine acceptable and unacceptable behavioral patterns among team members, in terms of their relationships to one another and their relationship to their work. Because a team is embedded within a larger organization, the team culture will usually include influences from and elements of the broader, overall organizational culture. But what makes it unique are the aspects of the team culture that are distinctive and not shared with the culture of the organization at large. For example, when a physician works with their team of other physicians, nurses, or healthcare providers, they may have shared experiences with a particular patient. These distinctive experiences may impact how the team interacts with that patient and with other patients. Those in the organization who do not share those experiences may not know the inside jokes and jargon that the team knows and uses to ensure consistent behavior among team members when engaging in team performance episodes (i.e., patient care processes).

A positive team culture is the shared set of values, beliefs, and attitudes that drives the development of positive team relationships, high productivity, flexibility, and adaptability (Willard-Grace et al., 2014). Joe was recently asked to facilitate a team meeting for a medical team that was struggling to perform well together. In the meeting, several things were observed, suggesting a negative, dysfunctional team culture. First, the leader did not take responsibility or really engage much at all (i.e., laissez-faire style). Second, the team members all tried to assert themselves, controlling the flow of patients, determining who works with which patient, and so forth (all likely Type A personalities). Third, conflict arose, and rather than a meaningful discourse of differing opinions, personal attacks emerged almost immediately. Joe then proceeded to educate the team in terms of the specific team strategies covered in Chapters 9 and 10, emphasizing that an engaged leader who provides needed direction and also fosters peer-to-peer collaboration will provide a better team experience for everyone. In other words, this was *not* an example of a positive team culture!

A positive team culture is established when a leader sets and communicates expectations that are achievable and inspiring; where team members know what it means to effectively collaborate (and do so); where person-ality and other form of diversity are embraced; where conflict is managed openly, directly, and constructively; and where accountability is shared by all and maintained by feedback (Shin et al., 2016). It takes effort on the part of both the leader and the team members to establish a positive team culture in the first place, and then the values, beliefs, and attitudes become shared, are positive, and create a team environment capable of achieving the benefits of the positive culture, which include reductions in stress, burnout, and, of course, error (Willard-Grace et al., 2014).

How to Establish a Positive Team Culture

The previous section defined organizational and team culture, and began to identify practices that can help to establish and maintain a positive team culture. Many of those behaviors were discussed in substantial detail in Chapters 9 and 10. Drawn from that content, we provide here by way of summary a list of six "do's" and five "don'ts" for creating a positive team culture. There are many such lists that can be easily found via your favorite search engine (e.g., Heinz, 2021); here we provide the strategies that are both readily available and scientifically supported by researchers and scholars working in these areas. The following list comprises those actions that we endorse and recommend based on our experience, available research, and current best practice. Thus, in summary, we provide our "prescriptions" for developing a positive team culture. For each "do" or "don't" we share an example from our observations in healthcare settings. We'll begin here with the do's.

1. *Do be clear on team goals.* Nothing motivates individuals and teams like a shared goal or problem to solve by the combined efforts of the team members (Van Mierlo & Van Hooft, 2020). Remember, teams exist to get things done, to accomplish important goals through coordinated action. Goal-setting theory is clear that when teams have an understanding of their shared purpose and goal, they are more engaged in their work and perform better (Locke & Latham, 1994). They tend to be happier and more effective as team members, because their efforts to collaborate match the shared desire to accomplish the team goal. The best, most motivating goals are those that are estab-lished collaboratively within the team. For example, if your clinic obtains patient satisfaction scores, collaboratively determine a specific rating you want to achieve together and then work hard to achieve it.

Perhaps you also want to increase the number of patients who complete the rating, so you have a more accurate picture of how you're doing. The key is to set goals together to the extent possible and then to work to achieve them together. If for whatever reason team goals cannot be set collaboratively, with full participation of all members, it is important that all fully understand the reason for the goal, why it is set, and what help or support can be accessed in order to help the team reach the goal. As much as the extensive literature on goal-setting indicates that full participation and collaboration are ideal in terms of promoting goal acceptance, many goals are set by management above the level of the team. When that is the case, it is essential that team members understand the "back story" so that they are willing to accept the goals and strive together to achieve them.

2. *Do promote diversity, inclusion, and respect.* All of us, as team leaders and members, want to feel included, to know that our diversity is valued and that mutual respect is assured, regardless of the differences among us (Pearson et al., 2007). One might boil this "do" down to playing nice, applying the iconic "kindergarten playground rules" (Fulghum, 2003). For many years, and especially recently, there has been a growing literature on the topic of team diversity and its benefits and risks. In most cases in medical teams (and teams in other HROs) there is a clear positional hierarchy. Such teams will automatically be diverse in terms of power, seniority, and other issues of privilege. There will be "natural" barriers to speaking up, especially questioning or challenging a superior. Those issues are best addressed by the leader, in setting the tone (and norms) for how the team will operate. But there is also diversity in background, gender, age, ethnicity, personality, nationality, and other factors. And the research clearly shows that teams that are diverse in terms of those demographics are ultimately more productive and creative, and even more cohesive, than those that are less diverse. We emphasize the key word "ultimately," as the research also shows that highly diverse teams are more likely to experience internal conflict early on ("storming") and may be slower to develop to their highest potential than more homogeneous teams. As our society has become more generally aware of the necessity of fostering inclusion, a team culture that embraces and celebrates diversity will thereby be a more positive culture.

3. *Do encourage and contribute to feedback.* Both team leaders and members need to encourage all team members to provide ongoing feedback to one another. Research is clear on the value of feedback within the

team. The data show consistently that feedback is one of the single most effective communication tools for teams to enhance motivation, satisfaction, and performance both in-person and virtually (Gabelica et al., 2012; Geister et al., 2006). Think of it this way. Goal-setting, as critically important as that is, is a kind of "ballistic shot"; we aim and release, and hope to hit the target. Ongoing feedback allows us to adapt and adjust as needed, in order to ensure that we actually do hit the target. Note too that feedback can be positive as well as corrective. Too often we think that feedback must always be critical, aimed at identifying and correcting problems, and although that is clearly one form of feedback, it is not the only type. Telling someone "good job" or "really great work today" is feedback as well, specifically, positive feedback. Nothing makes another physician's day more than to receive a compliment from a peer professional of whom they think highly. Just as there is an extensive research literature on goal-setting, there is also a great deal of published work on feedback. To boil down the most common themes, the data suggest strongly that feedback is most effective when it is frequent, accurate, specific, and timely. Indeed the acronym FAST is common in the feedback literature. "Frequent" captures the ongoing aspect. "Accurate" is essential. "Specific" is crucial, and often a missing element. So is "timely." Say a member of a medical team goes out of their way to calm a nervous and upset patient. Other team members may compliment that member as soon as possible after the event (timely), saying something like, "You were really supportive in taking the extra time to talk to that patient privately, and assure them of all the steps we were taking to ensure a safe and effective procedure" (accurate and specific). Giving this kind of feedback regularly within the team represents the "frequent" element. It is obviously more challenging to give corrective feedback, but especially if the FAST guidelines are followed, and deserved positive feedback is given as well as corrective feedback, the latter can and should be effective in redirecting behavior without damaging internal relationships within the team.

4. *Do be both transparent and flexible.* Being transparent when it comes to patient care should be a given. Open sharing of information about patients, their situation, their life, and so on may be essential in diagnosing and helping with care plans. Additionally, being transparent in professional needs or challenges from home that may be impacting work (or vice versa) is essential for maximum team effectiveness (Huffmeier et al., 2011). Essentially, this internal-team

transparency, requiring a high level of self-disclosure, initiates social support behavior on the part of others on the team. We have emphasized the critical impact of social support as a stress buffer, and obviously a positive team culture is a major source of just such support at work. Such social support may require additional flexibility on the part of other team members, to help another healthcare provider by, for example, picking up an extra patient in order to reduce their workload.

We recognize that self-disclosure can be very uncomfortable for many people, especially those who are more introverted, more Type A, or who are in positions of leadership and authority. Those characteristics apply to many in the healthcare enterprise, as we have discussed. As much as it might feel awkward and uncomfortable, high transparency within teams is nonetheless a marker of the most effective teams and, again, amplifies the social support "intervention," which the stress-management literature consistently highlights as so critically important. We must emphasize that trust is an essential foundation for the levels of transparency and self-disclosure that we are describing here.

5. *Do promote humor and social outings together.* Teams exist to get things done, but they are not "all work, only work." The team environment can and must include some degree of allowance for non-work-related social interaction, involving humor and joviality when appropriate (Tremblay, 2017). We recommend that team leaders and members embrace positive and uplifting humor within the team, and arrange and attend nonwork social occasions as simple as, for example, just going to lunch together and socializing. On a recent call with a primary care physician, Joe was talking about ways to optimize telehealth visits as a form of virtual meeting. In the conversation, the physician said, "Well, that should help make my telehealth visits better, but have you got anything to make my group work better together?" We were short on time, and so Joe simply suggested that they should eat lunch together. A few weeks later Joe got an unexpected call from this same physician who said, "How did you know that would work?" and Joe shared what you're reading here. Social outings, as simple as coffee or lunch, provide the opportunity for conversation, connection, humor, and empathy to grow.

Along similar lines, John's departmental meetings have a tradition of starting with "good news to share," which gives every team member an opportunity to talk about personal or professional accomplishments and to be celebrated by their peers. These meeting conclude with "as you like it," which gives team members to bring up any issues, personal or professional, that they want to share with the team. So, at the start and at the end of our business meetings, we take time for a mini "social outing" or "check in/out."

6. *Do remove barriers to success.* Professionals in all fields look for ways to improve their performance at their craft. Physicians and healthcare providers are no exception to this, and the National Institutes for Health and American Medical Association agrees that continuing medical education (CME) is of paramount importance (AMA Ed Hub, 2021). In addition to enabling each other to engage in CME, team leaders and members should help each other obtain additional training, adjust for work-schedule needs, and seek to remove any other barriers that may limit team effectiveness.

With all these positive behaviors in mind that both leaders and team members should engage in, the following is the list of "don'ts." As you might expect, many of them are fundamentally the opposite of the "do's."

1. *Don't engage in poor team management practices.* Basically, reread Chapter 9, practice all of those good team leader behaviors, and don't do the opposite! We state "management" practices here because physicians do not have to be defined, positional leaders to engage in management. After all, a physician has patients and they are primarily responsible for the management of their care and of those additional team members who assist in that care. Thus, a physician is a manager, and if they engage in poor management practices, it impacts their team members and their patients. Good management practices are a key to teamwork competency (Leggat, 2007). Thus, much of this "don't" is really just the opposite of the good advice in Chapter 9.

2. *Don't work through lunch.* It's important to have time to rest and recover to the extent possible during the workday, both psychologically and physically. Thus, we advise team leaders and team members to *not* skip lunch and work right through it, which is, unfortunately, an all too common practice. Instead, when possible, go to lunch together as a team (review Do #5). If going out to lunch is not possible in the time allotted, find a spot to eat the lunch you brought from home. Remember, this book is about burnout, and burnout is about being used up. Taking time for lunch is an opportunity to recharge your personal and team resources to finish the day strong.

A lunch break addresses both a biological need (i.e., a body needs fuel) and a psychological need. Take it! Sure, working through lunch could mean you finish your workday early or even just on time. But whatever you do that afternoon when you are at maybe 80 percent of your cognitive capacity will not be as effective as what you could do when you are at 100 percent. Given our focus on burnout and error, seems like 100 percent is a good idea.

3. *Don't limit learning opportunities.* Research on job demands and job engagement emphasizes the basic human need that people have to learn and grow (Chughtai & Buckley, 2011). For example, a nurse may want to learn how to do more of the tasks and duties associated with the work the physician is doing. If leaders give them the chance for some relevant on-the-job coaching and training (as opposed to informing them to "stay in their lane"), the nurse is likely to feel needed and valued, even more engaged in their job, and maybe even less likely to experience burnout. Simply stated, if a team member wants to learn something and it won't negatively impact the performance of their regular duties and responsibilities, there's no downside to encouraging learning.

4. *Don't hire clones of yourself.* In most physician and healthcare teams, full control over who is hired may not be within the team leaders/members' role and responsibility. But, as there are natural human tendencies to prefer to work with people who are like us, a bias to "hire more folks like us" can result in teams lacking in valuable diversity.

   Creating a team of homogeneous (i.e., all the same) folks can create barriers to innovation, creativity, and performance (Unsworth, 2001). In fact, there is strong, compelling evidence that having diversity within the team makes the team better in many ways, including performance, as we elaborated above (review Do #2). Thus, as team leaders and members, do embrace diversity and do not fall into the trap of hiring others based on their similarity to you.

5. *Don't inadvertently foster or allow disengagement.* For the many reasons we have addressed in this book, burnout is very likely to happen to healthcare team leaders and members from time to time. It is not 100 percent avoidable. When the symptoms occur, disengagement is often a natural response, indeed, one of the identifying facets of the burnout syndrome.. Thus, this "don't" is simple: when someone is showing signs of being burned out, leverage the positive team culture to bring the social support needed to reengage them. Otherwise, you

run the risk of normalizing disengagement, and disengagement does not help the physician, the team, or the patient, but only furthers the likelihood of burnout and error.

We are persuaded that team leaders and members who actively engage in these "do's" and avoid the "don'ts" will help establish and maintain a positive team culture. Although we have thus far spent the chapter explaining what culture is and how to create and sustain a good, positive one, you might wonder if all this effort is really worth it. The next section is all about *why* building a positive team culture is so essential to healthcare workers.

Exploring the Greater Benefits of a Positive Team Culture

A positive team culture is important for a variety of reasons. While in Chapter 10 we reviewed research on the benefits of teamwork and collaboration, there is additional research that addresses the broader issue of the positive team culture. Here we highlight some of the major findings from studies that assessed the overall culture of healthcare teams and identified positive outcomes that correlated with those assessments of team culture. First, according to Meterko and colleagues (2004), a positive teamwork culture in hospitals results in more positive experiences for patients. In fact, they found that a positive, highly collaborative teamwork culture was related to patients' positive experience, whereas a more rigid bureaucratic culture was negatively associated with patient satisfaction. A bureaucratic culture emphasizes the "red tape" so commonly found in healthcare settings, including the policies, procedures, and the forms (oh so many forms), which usually elicit a negative response from patients. Thus, a positive team culture is associated with positive relationships between the team and the patients.

Second, Shin and colleagues (2016) explored the relationship between team culture and both task performance and creative performance of healthcare teams. Using a sample of leaders and members of 104 teams, they found that team culture positively related to team task performance. In other words, teams with a more positive team culture that enables effective team processes tend to perform better than those that do not. In healthcare teams, team processes that promote better team performance mean better patient care, including fewer errors.

Third, and most important given the focus of this book, Willard-Grace and colleagues (2014) investigated the relationship between team culture in terms of the structure of teams and burnout. They found that a tight team structure was associated with less clinician burnout, particularly less of the contributing facet of exhaustion. Tight team structure in this study refers to the degree of overlap of roles as well the number of team members. Thus, having a smaller team whose members share roles and responsibilities to some extent results in reduced incidence of burnout.

Barriers to a Positive Team Culture

There is an important caution, though. Long-term teams that have established a positive culture run the risk of falling victim to "groupthink." That is, team members may so enjoy being on the team and supporting their leader that over time they become less willing to speak up and "disrupt the harmony of the team" if they disagree with the direction the team and its leader are taking. They self-censor, coming to value harmony and agreement over sound judgment. The extensive literature on groupthink includes a number of strategies for avoiding it. For example, the leader can set ground rules for respectful disagreement, thereby protecting the psychological safety of those who speak up and challenge, and team members may establish themselves as devil's advocates, with the role of taking the counterpoint and "testing" directions before they are taken.

Even in a short-term team, the leader may be so highly placed in the hierarchy (e.g., senior staff member, department head, top surgeon in the field) that team members may be intimidated even before coming together as a team. In such a situation, the leader can minimize groupthink by explicitly inviting team members to speak up, ask questions, or otherwise give information first, before the leader expresses their views. Such an invitation can include the statement that team members should all help each other and that the team cannot proceed unless everyone understands, agrees, has weighed the options, and commits to the action. It is critical that if someone does speak up, the leader acknowledges and appreciates the input. This "moment of truth" reinforces the message that input is welcomed and considered, and sets the tone for a team that collaborates rather than assuming "the boss knows what he's doing."

Summing Up

In sum, physicians and healthcare workers often work in teams. These teams can be optimized by building a positive team culture and through engaging in known best practices for team effectiveness, that is, critical "do's" and "don'ts." We advise team leaders and team members alike to seek to learn how to be better team members and help others develop the skills needed to be effective team members. The team then becomes a resource that can be leveraged to enhance performance and mitigate burnout for the entire team. Common barriers to developing and sustaining a positive team culture, including the risk of groupthink, while challenging, are not insurmountable.

The COVID-19 Effect

The coronavirus pandemic has also led to members of the health care team who may not normally work together to collaborate on crisis management. For example, emergency departments may have been repurposed as COVID-19 units, or new units temporarily assembled to deal with the sudden influx of patients. The pandemic required physicians and nurses to demonstrate a willingness to tackle challenges like never before, and often in teams they would never assemble during normal operations (Bourgault & Goforth, 2021). Teamwork had to emerge quickly and effectively to respond to the crisis. These teams learned to establish a healthy and positive team culture through consistent and authentic behaviors that help establish a healthy work environment. Thus, the effect of COVID-19 was to require instantaneous team forming and efficient team culture building; if not, a given healthcare system would never be able to accommodate the demands. From a team positive culture perspective, the COVID-19 effect was, in some cases, the enactment of the ideals shared in this chapter.

Key Takeaways

- Establishing and maintaining a positive team culture requires an eye toward the team composition challenges and opportunities within the work environment.
- Physicians as team leaders and team members have many things to do and not do to contribute to the building of the positive team culture.
- Groupthink is a major barrier to the development of a healthy and effective team culture and teamwork situation.

REFERENCES

AMA Ed Hub. (2021). Discover education from AMA, JN Learning™ (CME from the JAMA Network™) and more trusted sources – all in one place! https://edhub.ama-assn.org/pages/keep-current?gclid=CjwKCAjwieuGBhAs EiwA1Ly_nc-56ET5ZAqb7-pnNKgykoXTffy1xfE6-PzNefwro7tVJj7dUY Ue4hoCv1YQAvD_BwE.

Bourgault, A. M., & Goforth, C. (2021, June 1). Embrace teamwork to create and maintain a positive workplace culture. *Critical Care Nurse*, 41(3), 8–10.

https://aacnjournals.org/ccnonline/article/41/3/8/31452/Embrace-Teamwork-to-Create-and-Maintain-a-Positive.

Chughtai, A. A., & Buckley, F. (2011). Work engagement: Antecedents, the mediating role of learning goal orientation and job performance. *Career Development International, 16*(7), 684–705.

Fulghum, R. (2003). *All I Really Need to Know I Learned in Kindergarten: Reconsidered, Revised & Expanded with Twenty-Five New Essays.* New York: Random House Digital.

Gabelica, C., van den Bossche, P., Segers, M., & Gijselaers, W. (2012). Feedback, a powerful lever in teams: A review. *Educational Research Review, 7*(2), 123–144.

Geister, S., Konradt, U., & Hertel, G. (2006). Effects of process feedback on motivation, satisfaction, and performance in virtual teams. *Small Group Research, 37*(5), 459–489.

Heinz, K. (2021). What is work culture? How to build a positive environment. Builtin.com. Retrieved from https://builtin.com/company-culture/positive-work-culture.

Hüffmeier, J., & Hertel, G. (2011). Many cheers make light the work: How social support triggers process gains in teams. *Journal of Managerial Psychology, 26* (3), 185–204.

Leggat, S. G. (2007). Effective healthcare teams require effective team members: Defining teamwork competencies. *BMC Health Services Research, 7*(1), 1–10.

Locke, E. A., & Latham, G. P. (1994). Goal setting theory. *Motivation: Theory and Research, 13*, 29.

Meterko, M., Mohr, D. C., & Young, G. J. (2004). Teamwork culture and patient satisfaction in hospitals. *Medical Care*, 492–498.

Pearson, A., Srivastava, R., Craig, D., Tucker, D., Grinspun, D., Bajnok, I., ... & Gi, A. A. (2007). Systematic review on embracing cultural diversity for developing and sustaining a healthy work environment in healthcare. *International Journal of Evidence-Based Healthcare, 5*(1), 54–91.

Shin, Y., Kim, M., Choi, J. N., & Lee, S. H. (2016). Does team culture matter? Roles of team culture and collective regulatory focus in team task and creative performance. *Group & Organization Management, 41*(2), 232–265.

Tremblay, M. (2017). Humor in teams: Multilevel relationships between humor climate, inclusion, trust, and citizenship behaviors. *Journal of Business and Psychology, 32*(4), 363–378.

Unsworth, K. (2001). Unpacking creativity. *Academy of Management Review, 26* (2), 289–297.

Van Mierlo, H., & Van Hooft, E. A. (2020). Team achievement goals and sports team performance. *Small Group Research, 51*(5), 581–615.

Willard-Grace, R., Hessler, D., Rogers, E., Dubé, K., Bodenheimer, T., & Grumbach, K. (2014). Team structure and culture are associated with lower burnout in primary care. *The Journal of the American Board of Family Medicine, 27*(2), 229–238.

CHAPTER 12

Solution #8: Make Changes in Workflow in Organizations

I enjoy working with patients and seeing them become well. Patients are not the problem and volume of patients is really not the problem. To be honest, my biggest source of stress and burden that interrupts my evenings and weekends is EHR [electronic health records]. Something simply has to be done about that!

—Physician

You often see in the news things like "the growing healthcare crisis" and so forth. Often this is followed by statistics on how many people don't have insurance or the rising costs of insurance premiums. For me, it's finding enough trained physicians after losing yet another great person to burnout, depression, and in some cases, suicide!

—Hospital administrator

Our instructors warn us about burnout ... but they don't have any solutions.

—Medical student

The three poignant quotes above are drawn from our recent interviews with physicians, administrators, and medical students. The purpose in sharing them is to illustrate a shift in focus for this and the next few chapters. That is, solutions up to this point have focused on individual and team-level domains, where individuals, team leaders, and team members (and the culture of teamwork that they create) are the focus of the solutions. We now take a step beyond the individual and team levels and argue that much can and should be done at the organizational, professional society, and government levels. The burnout crisis is manifestly *not* simply an individual physician crisis, though it ultimately falls hardest on the individual healthcare provider. It's not even a crisis about teams of healthcare workers, powerful as that can be. This crisis involves individual organizations (e.g., hospitals), systems of healthcare, professional societies, and government agencies. Organizations can make stress-reduction efforts in their operating systems that individuals and even leaders of units may not be wholly enabled to do on their own (i.e., policy changes).

Similarly, there are broader systems-level changes that professional associations and governmental regulatory agencies, in their oversight role, can make to address the burnout crisis, to make it easier for hospitals and other medical practices, teams, and individuals to minimize their risk (Linzer et al., 2015).

This chapter begins exploring what we identify as "local" systems solutions by focusing specifically on workflow design and redesign at the organization level. Revisiting existing workflows and crafting more effective and efficient workflows is obviously beneficial to teams and individuals and, in most cases, is outside the direct control of individual physicians, their teams, and their direct team leaders.

Workflow in Healthcare Organizations

Analysis of workflow, or the processes through which work passes from initiation to completion, is obviously important in every industry, but is of particular interest and importance in the healthcare industry (Berg, 2019a). As the patient population continues to grow and age, efficient and effective workflow has become more and more critical to effective healthcare delivery. In healthcare, "workflow" refers to every step the patient encounters from entering to exiting the health service experience (e.g., AHRQ, 2021). Figure 12.1 illustrates how a typical noncritical, nonemergency patient moves through healthcare experiences: the patient enters the clinic or doctor's office, registers with administrative support staff, meets with a nurse, meets with a physician, may get laboratory work or other procedures done, gets results in a brief consultation, possibly gets prescriptions, settles up with billing/insurance, and then leaves. Note that in some cases these steps may not all be accomplished on the same day. Within each of these steps are smaller workflow steps followed by each individual who interacts with the patient. These include the protocols followed by the nurse when taking initial vitals, as well as the mental checklist of questions and processes that the physician follows during each exam and patient interaction (AHRQ, 2021).

Although all of this typical, generic workflow sounds both reasonable and effective, when bottlenecks in the process emerge, they can create frustration and stress that add to the risk of burnout (DeChant et al., 2019). Complete control over these processes is often out of the hands of any one physician, other medical professional, or the teams in which they

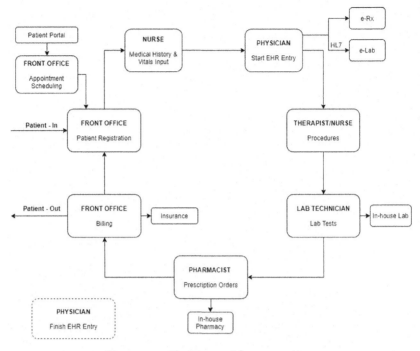

Figure 12.1   Physician workflow per patient.

work. Organizational policies, safety procedures, and laws (e.g., HIPAA), which set requirements and limits on what the local organizational system can do, govern and constrain some of the workflows within these interactions. While problems related to workflow may most strongly affect the "end-users" (i.e., physicians or other providers), and these healthcare providers can implement individual and team strategies to help reduce the associated stress, the long-term or ultimate solution or intervention must involve the organizational level. This is an absolutely critical point. As important as the individual and team-based solutions are, at the broader and more strategic level, the systems within which teams and individuals work (local systems, in our terms) must be designed for efficiency and effectiveness of use, and for the minimization of unnecessary and avoidable stress.

In a recent systematic review of organization-directed workplace interventions to address physician burnout, four domains of interventions were identified: (1) teamwork initiatives (addressed in detail in Chapters 9–11); (2) time initiatives focused on duty hour restrictions; (3) transitions, referring to workflow changes via policy adjustments; and (4) technology-related interventions, mostly centered around electronic health records (EHR; DeChant et al., 2019). The results of this review suggested that the greatest burnout reduction occurs in relation to the latter two initiatives, namely, workflow changes and technology improvements and changes, especially reducing the burden of EHR. In practice, these two initiatives are intimately connected. Often a workflow change would involve a change in how and to what extent physicians or others are engaged in nonclinical, tech-related activities. Specifically, adjustments that impacted the time spent on certain nonclinical, administrative tasks had the largest impact on physician burnout, consistent with the data we presented in Chapter 2.

In an article on the same topic commissioned by the American Medical Association (Berg, 2019b), implementation of the four specific workflow strategies outlined below were shown to cut burnout risk by 45 percent.

1. *Call management.* A typical phone call into a doctor's office or clinic was dealt with by an average of seven different individuals before being resolved. Instead, consider a "one-touch" goal, meaning to resolve the call by the first person who takes it or listens to the message – that is, have one central point of contact. In most cases, such a change would require expanded training for the central contact individual, and a higher level of authority than is typical for receptionists, accounts management personnel, and other administrative support personnel.

2. *Inbox management.* If responding promptly to incoming calls, emails, regular mail, and other contacts presents a challenge, consider hiring an additional nurse practitioner to cover physicians' "inboxes" when they are seeing patients. Such a change would allow doctors to spend more time with patients (always a concern), and thus would allow patients to receive a quicker response to their concerns. It would also reduce inbox work after hours by physicians and others, which is widely seen as a burden and source of stress.

3. *Decompressed clinic schedules.* Create time within the day for physicians to do documentation by inserting "administrative" time in their schedule. This is admittedly quite challenging when doctors are operating on a fee-for-service, volume-based business model, which encourages maximizing the number of patients seen. We will have much more to say about this prevailing model later.

4. *Share the care.* Put the responsibility of clinic flow and workflow on the people at the ground level, where solutions can be identified and

implemented quickly. Again, this strategy would involve additional training and expanded authority for all members of the team, including physicians' assistants, nurses, and administrative assistants.

It should be noted that these interventions could – and likely would – address one of the main concerns captured in an opening quote to this chapter. Maintaining EHR presents a considerable time burden to physicians, especially as there are certain physician-specific tasks in updating EHR, that is, tasks that cannot be delegated to nurses or assistants. For example, in an opinion article in 2018, Downing and colleagues discussed the crisis of burnout and pointed to EHR as a major driver of that burnout. Then, in 2020, a study by Anderson, Leubner, and Brown analyzed the after-hours time spent by family physicians on HER-related work. They found that physicians spent an average of 4.5 hours per month in addition to regular working hours on EHR, with some physicians spending as much as 33 hours per month. Thus, even though EHR is not the only driver of burnout, it is yet another demand placed on an already stressed system of physicians. Therefore, decompressed clinic schedules or other mechanisms to assist with EHR may show the greatest reductions in physician burnout, at least from a workflow perspective. But again, the prevailing business model for many doctors makes the prospect of reducing patient panels especially challenging.

In sum, the recommended means to reduce physician and healthcare provider burnout at the local system level are to implement changes in workflow, reduce the number of hand-offs, eliminate or at least minimize pinch points, and, overall, streamline the work of providing healthcare services (Hung et al., 2018). However, because these common workflows are often policy-driven and controlled at the organization level, system administrators and organizational leaders would need to take the initiative to push these efforts forward and advocate for them. Consistent with Hung and colleagues' recommendations, consider the following "how to" steps that organizational leaders could take to streamline workflows:

1. *Discover the workflow issue.* First, conduct a "current-state" analysis. Talk to physicians and other healthcare providers in your system in order to do the homework needed to understand the workflow issue and the extent to which it is a problem within the organization/ system. As is done in other industries, a front-door to back-door, step-by-step analysis finds pinch points, bad hand-offs, and other inefficiencies that have developed over time "on their own" and, once identified, can be engineered out. In the healthcare setting, a thorough

workflow analysis should be undertaken to identify when and how a patient first makes contact with the system, who "touches" them, what they do with them, what happens next, and who is involved, all the way through to completion of the healthcare delivery process.

2. *Seek recommendations from the ground level.* In addressing step 1 above, involve the physicians, nurses, and all others within your patient workflow process and ask them to recommend changes they believe might make a difference. The people closest to the problem are surely the ones thinking most about it, and the ones who may well have the best ideas. They are the internal subject matter experts, and their hands-on experience is invaluable in conducting a workflow analysis. Additionally, it can be helpful to seek a professional with expertise in workflow and redesign and incorporate their recommendations. As a sidenote, John and Joe have been called upon as outside "experts" to oversee workflow analyses in several industries. In every case, without exception, we have found inefficiencies that could be (and were) corrected. Again, workflows for the most part grow organically; their growth is rarely planned and managed effectively.

3. *Invite and deploy a team to change/revise/adjust policies.* Collaboratively changing policy will make the changes much more adaptable by those most impacted by the change. Allow a team of internal subject matter experts, a design team, to work together (again, perhaps assisted by an outside professional) to propose the new policies.

4. *Implement changes following the best pre- and postintervention assessment practices.* Implement the changes but do so in a way that allows for measurement before, during, and after the implementation. After all, what good is an intervention that cannot be objectively shown to reduce the risk of burnout and enhance efficiency and effectiveness at the same time? And when the changes in workflow are implemented, understand that conditions change over time, and today's improvement may become tomorrow's inefficiency. So, the process of assessing and adapting workflow cannot be a one-off; it must be an ongoing process.

Worth emphasizing is the fact that effective workflow interventions have the side benefit of building individual engagement, enhancing teamwork, and improving overall operational effectiveness. When an organization is willing to invest the time and effort needed to improve work processes, that investment sends a strong and positive message to employees of the organization: "They care.... They want to make things easier for us....

They hear us, and act on our suggestions." Thus, while truly addressing burnout and the risks associated with it, other desirable outcomes may also be achieved as a result of changing workflows in a positive way.

Barriers to Proposed Solutions

There are two major barriers to the proposed workflow-improvement solutions that deserve mention here. First is the requisite buy-in from the top management team in healthcare systems and the related resources they provide. Those seeking to make such a change must convince local healthcare leadership at the appropriate decision-making level that things need to change and help them identify the strategies and tools to make lasting change. In most cases, the broad metrics provided in this text (e.g., EHR after hours) may serve as a useful argument for convincing decision makers to initiate change and avert further problems. However, it may be essential to be proactive and provide data from one's own locale to justify resource allocation to the cause. The second major barrier is actually convincing the physicians and healthcare providers themselves to change their behavior once the workflow adjustments are implemented. As in all workplace environments, one of the major barriers to behavioral change is the traditions and rhythms of the old ways of doing things (Lavoie et al., 2017). Any intervention that will change workflows will require changing how things have always been done in favor of what may be better, and trial and error processes may come into play. Thus, getting physicians to buy into the changes and give them a try will be essential.

The COVID-19 Effect

Major crises always bring change, during and after the crisis. The more intense and severe the crisis, the greater the magnitude of the change and the greater the rate at which it occurs. As but one of many examples of the system-level impact of a major crisis, World War I inspired the launch of the mental testing movement, as the US military had to quickly assess the abilities of many thousands of recruits. The "Army Alpha" and "Army Beta" were developed very quickly. Intelligence tests had been developed earlier for children, for example, the Binet-Simon tests and the US English adaptation, the Stanford-Binet test, but they were not widely used. That all changed during the war, and the aptitude testing movement continues today, with tests like the SAT, ACT, GRE, MCAT, LSAT, and many more.

The pandemic is a crisis of similar magnitude. Suddenly, a major, unexpected global healthcare crisis was unleashed on the world, triggering a devastating economic crisis as well. During the peak of a crisis, the challenge is survival. Strategies and tactics, from the systems level on down are put in place to keep us safe and secure, to the extent possible. People long for a "return to normal." But after the peak of the crisis, when things stabilize, there is never a full-on return to the old normal. Some of the short-term changes persist, and some elements of the "old normal" no longer fit.

As much as no one wished for the pandemic, it is causing us to rethink many aspects of our lives. This is true in healthcare, to be sure. Which policies and procedures of the past should be changed, and how? Which stop-gap policies and procedures during the peak should be maintained? Which new policies and procedures, protocols, management strategies, best practices should be put in place?

This is the time for a "reset." All our research, including the published studies that we have reviewed and the data gathered through our interviews, points clearly to the problems with the systems that have evolved over the last several decades. Government programs, regulatory constraints, common policies, procedures, and protocols have collectively had the unintended consequence of adding to the stress level of healthcare professionals, and thus increasing the risk of burnout. As much as the individual and team solutions we have proposed are beneficial, and should be practiced, they allow doctors and other providers to make the best of a bad situation. The ultimate "fix" has to be at the systems level. It has to be top-down.

Decades ago, there was a push for "total quality" in US manufacturing. Researchers argued that quality problems were not due to uncaring workers or poor teamwork, but instead were due to poor systems that made it virtually inevitable that scrap would be produced and rework would be required. Assembly-line production systems often added error, which teams and individual workers could not completely avoid or offset. The battle cry of the total quality management movement was, "Change the systems!"

And so it is, we contend, with healthcare. During and even before the pandemic, doctors and others are working in archaic systems that have been designed and implemented piecemeal, virtually guaranteeing added stress and burnout risk.

We were taught many years ago that the Chinese character for "crisis" translates as "dangerous opportunity." The opportunity delivered by the pandemic can and should include redesigning healthcare systems for effectiveness and efficiency, minimizing the stress of the job (there is plenty there already), and reducing the risk of burnout.

Futurist Joel Barker said that a paradigm shift resets everything to zero. His point was that when there is a major disruption, a quantum shift, past practice doesn't guarantee anything about the present or the future. We all have the opportunity, even the requirement, to rethink things.

The pandemic has brought a paradigm shift in healthcare, to be sure. When we can catch our breath, the question will be which "systems" factors no longer make sense, and which new policies do. Government regulators, CEOs of healthcare systems, managers of hospitals, and physicians in private practice, as well as nurses, physicians' assistants, pharmacists, and all others in the chain of events in healthcare delivery should be examining the systems in which they work, and recommending and making adaptive changes in their approach to caring for patients.

Key Takeaways

- Some solutions to the burnout crisis are largely within the control of the leaders of local healthcare systems, and can and should be implemented.
- One such systems-issue is workflow analysis and workflow improvement. It is within the authority of local leadership to engage employees and outside experts to review and streamline the "steps in the process" of providing their healthcare services.
- One of the unintended consequences of the coronavirus pandemic is that, as with all major crises, it has provided the opportunity, even the necessity, to broadly rethink how we do things. As much as no one would have ever wished for this health and economic disaster, it will give systems leaders at every level the platform for making major change, if they choose to do so. The post-pandemic world will not be a simple return to business as usual, lapsing back into healthcare systems requirements that necessarily trigger burnout. Many things will be very different. Healthcare delivery can and should be rethought and reset.

REFERENCES

AHRQ. (2021). Flowchart. Digital Healthcare Research. https://digital.ahrq.gov/health-it-tools-and-resources/evaluation-resources/workflow-assessment-health-it-toolkit/all-workflow-tools/flowchart.

Anderson, J., Leubner, J., & Brown, S. (2020). EHR overtime: An analysis of time spent after hours by family physicians. *Family Medicine*, *52*(2), 135–137.

Berg, S. (2019a). Physician burnout: The pledge your organization should make now. AMA Physician Health. Retrieved from www.ama-assn.org/practice-management/physician-health/physician-burnout-pledge-your-organization-should-make-now.

(2019b). These 4 workflow changes help cut burnout by 45%. AMA Physician Health. Retrieved from www.ama-assn.org/practice-management/physician-health/these-4-workflow-changes-help-cut-burnout-45.

DeChant, P. F., Acs, A., Rhee, K. B., Boulanger, T. S., Snowdon, J. L., Tutty, M. A., Sinsky, C. A., & Thomas Craig, K. J. (2019). Effect of organization-directed workplace interventions on physician burnout: A systematic review. *Mayo Clinic Proceedings. Innovations, Quality & Outcomes*, *3*(4), 384–408. https://doi.org/10.1016/j.mayocpiqo.2019.07.006.

Downing, N. L., Bates, D. W., & Longhurst, C. A. (2018). Physician burnout in the electronic health record era: Are we ignoring the real cause? *Annals of Internal Medicine*, *169*(1), 50–51. https://doi.org/10.7326/M18-0139.

Hung, D. Y., Harrison, M. I., Truong, Q., & Du, X. (2018). Experiences of primary care physicians and staff following lean workflow redesign. *BMC Health Services Research*, *18*(1), 274.

Lavoie, K. L., Rash, J. A., & Campbell, T. S. (2017). Changing provider behavior in the context of chronic disease management: Focus on clinical inertia. *Annual Review of Pharmacology and Toxicology*, *57*, 263–283.

Linzer, M., Poplau, S., Grossman, E., Varkey, A., Yale, S., Williams, E., . . . & Kohnhorst, D. (2015). A cluster randomized trial of interventions to improve work conditions and clinician burnout in primary care: Results from the Healthy Work Place (HWP) study. *Journal of General Internal Medicine*, *30*(8), 1105–1111.

CHAPTER I 3

Solution #9: Make Changes in Management Practices in Local Healthcare System Top Leaders

> They call it the "great resignation." For my people, it's not the great resignation, but the "great burnout"!
>
> —Hospital administrator

That comment came from a hospital administrator frustrated by the mass departure of so many physicians and nurses from the ranks as a result, in part, of the workload and death witnessed during the coronavirus pandemic. In addition to the group leadership solutions discussed in the previous chapter centered on workflow analysis and workflow streamlining, there are a variety of management-driven practices that local healthcare system leaders can and should consider in their effort to reduce stress and the risk of burnout for their healthcare employees. Interestingly, these practices mirror the previously discussed solutions around individual, team, leader, and organization strategies. One might conclude, rightly, that there are essentially two approaches: bottom-up (discussed in the previous chapters) and top-down (discussed in this and the next two chapters). Bottom-up refers to solution approaches that target the people doing the work at the bottom of the organizational hierarchy such as physicians and nurses, who meet directly with patients. Top-down refers to solution approaches, like the one discussed in this chapter, which target decision makers at the top leadership/management level of the organization, such as CEOs and other top administrators of healthcare systems. While perhaps simplistic, this bottom-up/top-down dichotomy does capture much of the essence of the solutions discussed throughout this book. However, in order for most of the efforts to be implemented holistically across a local healthcare system, CEOs of these systems and leaders at all levels must act together.

What Are Top Management Roles in Healthcare?

We often use the terms "manager" and "leader" interchangeably, but they are not the same. "Manager" is a position in the organizational hierarchy.

168

A manager has direct-report employees, for whom the manager ideally provides direction and support. A leader is someone who inspires others to follow their vision, their strategy, to work toward shared goals. "Leader" is not per se a position in the hierarchy. One can be a leader without being a (positional) manager. One can be a manager without being an (inspirational) leader. One of the reasons the two terms are so often conflated is that, ideally, a manager (with power of position) is also a leader (with the ability to influence and inspire). Although management and leadership are not always intertwined, there are a number of positions or roles in healthcare management that lend themselves to the kinds of leadership needed to make a large-scale impact on burnout among physicians and healthcare workers. The top five healthcare management jobs include hospital CEO, hospital/healthcare CFO, hospital/healthcare administrator, pharmaceutical product manager, and medical practice manager (Utica College, 2021). In general, one would consider the first three on that list as "top management"/executive, while the other two would be more "mid-level management." Regardless, these roles typically involve substantial control over resources, as well as a major impact on policies, procedures, and practices within their respective organizations or local healthcare systems. For example, a hospital/healthcare administrator is often involved with hiring and firing decisions, though the actual act of hiring or firing may be delegated to an HR representative. In fact, the head of HR may also be making hiring or firing decisions as well, which introduces another manager into the mix. Additionally, all of these roles impact the strategic planning and operations of the organization. As such, these roles have a disproportionate impact on the day-to-day experiences of physicians and therefore have the potential for dramatic impact on the implementation of all the previous solutions discussed in this book, as well as the others we discuss here and in subsequent chapters.

Best Practices in Healthcare Management

Within these executive positions, organizations that train future health services administrators and leaders have identified some traits or actions for effective leadership in healthcare (University of Wyoming, 2021). These seven prescriptions, which frankly are pretty obvious, could easily be applied to most leadership roles, including those we have addressed in previous chapters. For the most part, they have universal application for successful leadership, but we bring them up here with a focus and emphasis on leadership in healthcare, particularly those top-level executives who have the greatest impact on the workings of physicians and other healthcare workers. We present the "healthcare management best practices" prescriptions here.

1. *Be curious.* This simple prescription refers to learning about new and innovative tools that you can get your hands on as well as being willing to consider new ways of doing things. Obviously, healthcare practice evolves and improves over time as new technology, tools, and procedures emerge. Stay abreast of those things and be willing to let those you lead try them. The new ways of doing things may hold the key to mitigating burnout, to some degree. It is important to be mindful, though, that "new ways" such as EHR can have unintended consequences that can have the opposite of the intended effect.

2. *Rely on the data.* Allow the data being collected in the organization be your guide to decision-making. Too often decisions are made based more on a "gut feeling" than on an accurate and unbiased interpretation of the hard data. The data can obviously provide factual inputs to decisions and can provide a defense against challengers to a given decision. Throughout this book we have cited many studies to indicate that our advice is drawn from the best available research. Similarly, this prescription simply says look to the data, the best available data, and the best current interpretation of those data, in making decisions.

3. *Set expectations.* Leaders in healthcare need to be specific about the challenges their people are facing, to seek desired solutions, to lead in a fair decision-making process, and to set the vision for the organization. Setting and communicating vision and mission, and related strategic plans, allows for setting and communicating relevant performance and teamwork expectations, and ultimately for holding people fairly accountable for meeting those expectations. Depending on what those expectations are and how they are enacted, a healthy work culture (or an unhealthy one) will emerge. Thus, fair expectations, clearly communicated and embraced by all, can become a tool in mitigating burnout.

4. *Lead by example.* If a leader expects people to do or not to do something, they themselves must act in accordance with their expectation. For example, if a physician leader expects people to have work-family balance by not engaging in EHR off hours, then the log should clearly show that they themselves are not logging in to update records on Sunday night at 10 p.m. (unless that's their shift). Overall, leading

by example means not being hypocritical, not violating your own expectations for others. No "rules for thee but not for me."

5. *Be dedicated to self-improvement.* Because healthcare is constantly changing, leaders need to be constantly learning. Continuing medical education is not just for the people directly interacting with patients. Leaders in healthcare need to be committed to their own self-improvement by engaging in continuing medical education that will allow them to assist in the identification of opportunities for greater efficiencies and greater effectiveness. (This best-practice prescription overlaps with #1.)

6. *Be adaptable.* If 2020 taught us one thing, it's the need to be flexible in crisis situations. As we have emphasized at the end of each chapter, COVID-19 has made healthcare adapt in ways the enterprise was largely unprepared for. Thus, effective leaders in healthcare must be adaptable and willing to make changes to their organization and for all those who work therein as needs and situations change.

7. *Communicate, communicate, communicate.* A common thread throughout all these best practices is the need to communicate them to everyone in the leader's organization. Further, other than not setting an expectation at all, nothing is worse than setting an expectation, not communicating it, and then wondering why no one is achieving the expected outcomes. Thus, it is important to communicate, to listen for feedback, and to be willing to do all the things previously listed as needed in response to the feedback.

Although these best-practice behaviors are identified as essential for effective leaders, too many do not apply them. However, as leaders do enact these strategies, they become able to engage in the solutions that we address next, namely, actions that directly reduce the risk of burnout.

Healthcare System Leaders and Burnout Reduction

In 2016, a group of ten CEOs of large local healthcare systems met at the American Medical Association (AMA) headquarters in Chicago to discuss how to respond to the burnout crisis plaguing their respective organizations (Noseworthy et al., 2017). In addition to reviewing much of the hard data that are also summarized in this book, they identified several things that they would collectively do at their respective institutions and beyond, to help respond to the crisis. We summarize their planned actions and expound on them relative to the responsibilities of leaders in these healthcare environments. The actions are divided into those actions that they can take directly at their institutions (things they can do) and advocacy actions for changes beyond their immediate control (things they can recommend).

Direct Immediate Actions for Healthcare Leaders

1. *Survey physician well-being on a regular basis and include a well-being measure as a critical performance measure for the institution.* Most organizations (74 percent as of August 2020), including hospitals, do an engagement survey (Wiles, 2020). The purpose of these surveys is generally to find out the extent to which employees are engaged at work, and to identify ways to build higher levels of engagement, because all the data show that a more engaged workforce is a high-performing workforce (Mackay et al., 2017). Although that is true, these annual surveys often miss the mark when it comes to identifying key factors that can reduce engagement. Most do not include burnout as a specific topic for consideration, and even fewer consider work-family balance issues, or any number of other issues we've already discussed in relation to the causes of burnout. However, healthcare leaders need to get data on staff well-being as a first step to help them make targeted decisions that will help physicians mitigate the risk of burnout.
2. *Quantify the financial costs of losing physicians as a result of burnout and other causes.* In addition to measuring the well-being of physicians and healthcare workers, including assessing burnout, healthcare leaders should undertake an assessment of the financial costs of losing physicians and determine the role that burnout plays in their turnover. What are their HR staff learning from exit interviews with doctors who leave? We have a pretty good guess. In 2020 the *New York Times* posted an article about how physicians are leaving their practices during the coronavirus pandemic, citing stress and burnout as a major factor (Abelson, 2020). As the pandemic abates, the need for primary care physicians and specialists at all levels will resume, and an already strapped system will likely feel an even greater burden. Getting the data on the cost of losing and replacing physicians and other healthcare workers, combined with the data on burnout-related turnover, will surely justify and defend decisions to implement any number of the solutions we have proposed.
3. *Encourage physicians and administrators to develop their leadership skills, build teamwork, and reduce the burden of administrative/nonclinical*

tasks that contribute to burnout. Frankly, this one could be boiled down to "read the previous four chapters and *do it!*" In other words, with the data in hand, all the measures that can be taken to act on the problem are there. The key here is policy changes that healthcare leaders can support and enact directly. A prime example elaborated in the previous chapter includes adjusting workflows to eliminate bottlenecks and pinch points in the healthcare delivery process and minimizing the burden of nonclinical tasks. In the course of interviews with a large group of physicians, Dillon and colleagues (2019) discovered once again that the EHR burden is perceived as wearing out physicians. Thus, it is essential to figure out ways to change how the system operates, write the policies to then make those changes, and enforce them.

Advocacy and Indirect Actions for Healthcare Leaders

1. *Educate peers in leadership positions to support research aimed at identifying policies to reduce burnout and promote wellness among physicians and other healthcare professionals.* As a leader engages in immediate actions of the type identified here that are under their control, they also have an opportunity to become advocates for strategies that are not under their control but are instead enacted by others. Thus, leaders need to engage with their network, share their successes and failures, and support the research to identify and establish effective policies across the healthcare enterprise. In essence, leaders need to cultivate a community of peer leaders to align the values to the desired, burnout- mitigating culture and provide resources to those on the front lines to do the things necessary to make a difference (Shanafelt & Noseworthy, 2017). Selfishly, John and Joe would love to see more funds flow from healthcare leaders to researchers to pilot-test any of a wide range of interventions that could support policies in healthcare for mitigating physician burnout. However, many of the solutions at the local systems level simply need leaders to jointly engage and put their collective heads together and act. That's what advocacy in this area means: collaboratively promoting the solutions through policy change.

2. *Work through the American Medical Association and similar national organizations to gather and disseminate best practices from institutions that have developed programs and policy changes that help reduce burnout and promote wellness.* Other HROs have developed just the sort of incident-capturing and best-practice dissemination processes that are

identified here. In the case of healthcare, the AMA is well positioned to provide such a service. In fact, the AMA in the United States and the British Medical Association in the United Kingdom curate websites full of best-practice strategies for more effectively managing burnout, and we have cited many of their available resources throughout the book.

3. *Encourage and support the American Medical Association and similar national organizations in influencing the government to reduce the regulatory burden, including the burden of EHR, which is known to add substantially to the burnout risk for healthcare providers.* In addition, encourage regulators and technology vendors to align the technology more closely with advanced models of team-based healthcare.

Healthcare leaders need to begin to see themselves as some of the more powerful members of a larger community within the overall healthcare system. That system is regulated by local and national governments. Thus, to the degree that a leader is allowed, they could be supporting national organizations such as the AMA and the BMA in their efforts to lobby legislatures, governors, presidents, and other national leaders to support laws and regulations that enable healthcare providers to reduce workload burdens and help control the burnout crisis. As mentioned previously, an unintended consequence of meaningful regulations around healthcare records was the EHR crisis and burden (HIPAA Journal, 2021). Now that we see the consequences of that regulation, national organizations and governmental leaders need to feel the pressure from healthcare leaders to address this challenge and other external pressures on physicians that contribute to burnout.

Barriers and Opportunities

On discovering the article that laid out the recommendations of the 2016 meeting of ten top CEOs in healthcare, we must admit we were surprised, initially somewhat heartened by their clear commitment and call to action, but, finally, somewhat concerned. We were pleasantly surprised and heartened to see that many of the items on this list speak to the very solutions discussed within this book. Further, the solutions recommended by the top executives who were surveyed acknowledge the critical need for leadership at the highest levels of the local healthcare systems to achieve change – again, top-down – acknowledging that there are limits to what an individual can do, working within systems created by others, to which they must accommodate. Additionally, the leaders noted that this is a problem that is significant enough to warrant work at the national and international levels. We encourage any CEOs and other leaders in local healthcare systems to commit to these same tasks and activities within their respective areas, with the expectation that the top-down approach may prove not only useful but essential to creating lasting change in physician and healthcare provider burnout.

The source of our disappointment is that this excellent set of recommendations was developed more than five years ago, and the problems identified as contributing to the burnout crisis continue today, no less than before and, indeed, more so. As we have noted throughout this book, the burnout problem not only persists but is growing. While sensible remedial actions have been widely recommended, they have not consistently been put into place.

Further, there are a several additional components to a comprehensive solution that can originate with healthcare system leaders. First, remember the importance of a collaborative approach involving physicians, nurses, and healthcare providers at all levels when implementing changes in policies, procedures, and practices. Throughout the discussion of implementing the strategies proposed in this chapter, the idea of collaboration between leadership and health system members was essentially assumed. But team science would be unwilling to simply assume collaboration, and would rather acknowledge the need to intentionally bring all relevant parties to the table for discussions of changes that need to be made. Our recommendation is to always emphasize a collaborative approach in any top-led effort. Effective system-level changes are always led from the top, but not in isolation. Leaders who can transform parts or all of their organization must seek input and engagement from the people who must enact the changes. They lead, but they collaborate with others.

Personal accountability and responsibility are essential for any collaborative initiative aimed at implementing the solutions that are presented in these chapters. However, in most cases, as we know, physicians, nurses, and other healthcare providers are already busy, and many are overwhelmed. The same may very well be true for most leaders in local healthcare systems. To achieve meaningful change with accountability and responsibility, someone or some group must be tasked with spearheading the initiatives. Some have argued that the appointment of an executive-level chief wellness officer at major healthcare organizations is needed (Shanafelt & Sinsky, 2020). This individual would have the responsibility to carry out the initiatives, hold those involved accountable, and take responsibility for the successes and failures in promoting physician health and well-being within the healthcare system.

In fact, the American Medical Association (Shanafelt & Sinsky, 2020) assembled a chief wellness officer (CWO) road map that includes advice to new CWOs. Specifically, they provided a nine-step strategy for leading change as a wellness officer as follows: (1) Clearly define your scope and charge; (2) study and understand your organization; (3) build your team; (4) identify existing organizational programs, gaps, and resources; (5) define and develop your team's mission and strategy; (6) establish partnerships, distributed leadership, and thematic task forces; (7) develop bidirectional communication strategy; (8) set performance metrics for the organization and the team; and (9) avoid common pitfalls and mistakes. Because of the benefits that have already emerged for local healthcare systems across the United States, the Collaborative for Healing and Renewal in Medicine CWO Network was formed with the purpose of providing a community of CWO leaders who can help each other navigate the challenging landscape of improving the health and well-being of healthcare providers (Shanafelt et al., 2020). Thus, our concluding recommendation is to hire and empower a champion for change in every healthcare system in the United States, United Kingdom, and beyond.

Summing Up

In sum, Solution #9 is really about obtaining buy-in from healthcare system leadership, collaboratively implementing the proposed solutions that they directly control, lobbying for those beyond their direct control, and providing adequate resources in terms of personnel and time to implement, evaluate, and assess the impact of the efforts. Because of the multifaceted nature of the problem and the need for coordination and collaboration throughout, our ultimate recommendation is to hire executive-level CWOs. These leaders can form the team to lead the charge within a given healthcare system. Yet again, since conditions change over time, sometimes rapidly, solutions led by local healthcare systems leaders must be flexible and adaptable, revisited as needed.

The COVID-19 Effect

Physician burnout was a recognized occupational syndrome and a cause of suboptimal patient care long before the coronavirus hit. During that time, there were calls for system-level interventions to improve physician well-being, including the appointment of leaders to champion the well-being initiatives, such as CWOs (Shanafelt et al., 2020). During the pandemic, CWOs quickly learned important lessons regarding how healthcare organizations can best address workforce well-being, even during a global crisis. CWOs identified evolving sources of worker anxiety, deployed support resources, participated in operational decision-making, and assessed the impact of fluid pandemic protocols on physician well-being. In other words, they continued to implement management practices designed to mitigate physician burnout. As the pandemic begins to become more manageable, healthcare organizations and their CWOs must attend to the well-being of the workforce by incorporating well-being management protocols into ongoing system processes in order to build and sustain a resilient healthcare workforce.

Key Takeaways

- All healthcare leaders need to learn about and engage in healthcare management best practices. This ensures that the leaders are the exemplars of care for their physicians.
- Healthcare leaders must take immediate action to quantify the costs of burnout among their physicians and encourage their healthcare workforce to develop the knowledge and skills to address the ongoing burnout issue.
- Healthcare leaders are uniquely positioned to be the advocates for change, including simple education and training for all physicians and healthcare workers.
- Healthcare system leadership should consider identifying and hiring a chief wellness officer to champion initiatives identified through the process of learning what is needed in their respective local healthcare systems.

REFERENCES

Abelson, R. (2020, November 15). Doctors are calling it quits under stress of the pandemic. *New York Times*. www.nytimes.com/2020/11/15/health/Covid-doctors-nurses-quitting.html.

Dillon, E. C., Tai-Seale, M., Meehan, A., Martin, V., Nordgren, R., Lee, T., Nauenberg, T., & Frosch, D. L. (2019). Frontline perspectives on physician burnout and strategies to improve well-being: Interviews with physicians and health system leaders. *Journal of General Internal Medicine, 35*(1), 261–267. https://doi.org/10.1007/s11606-019-05381-0.

HIPAA Journal. (2021). What is the HITECH Act? *HIPAA Journal.* www .hipaajournal.com/what-is-the-hitech-act/.

Mackay, M. M., Allen, J. A., & Landis, R. S. (2017). Investigating the incremental validity of employee engagement in the prediction of employee effectiveness: A meta-analytic path analysis. *Human Resource Management Review, 27*(1), 108–120. https://doi.org/10.1016/j.hrmr.2016.03.002.

Noseworthy, J. (2017). Physician burnout is a public health crisis: A message to our fellow health care CEOs. Health Affairs.org. Retrieved from www .healthaffairs.org/do/10.1377/hblog20170328.059397/full/.

Shanafelt, T., Farley, H., Wang, H., & Ripp, J. (2020, November). Responsibilities and job characteristics of health care chief wellness officers in the United States. *Mayo Clinic Proceedings, 95*(11), 2563–2566.

Shanafelt, T. D., & Noseworthy, J. H. (2017). Executive leadership and physician well-being: Nine organizational strategies to promote engagement and reduce burnout. Paper presented at the Mayo Clinic Proceedings.

Shanafelt, T. D., & Sinsky, C. A. (2020, June 25). Chief wellness officer road map. AMA Ed Hub. https://edhub.ama-assn.org/steps-forward/module/ 2767764.

University of Wyoming MS in Health Services Administration. Top 7 best practices in healthcare management. (2021, January 13). www .uwyohealthadminms.org/blog/healthcare-management-best-practices/.

Utica College. (2021). The top five healthcare management jobs. Utica College Online. https://programs.online.utica.edu/articles/top-five-healthcare-man agement-jobs.

Wiles, J. (2020). 9 questions that should be in every employee engagement survey. Smarter with Gartner. www.gartner.com/smarterwithgartner/the-9- questions-that-should-be-in-every-employee-engagement-survey/.

CHAPTER 14

Solution #10: Make Changes in Overall Healthcare System Processes

> For years we talked about [physician] burnout. We even did resiliency training. Now that it's here, and COVID, am I too late? Perhaps. But, I gotta try.
>
> —Hospital administrator

While our previous chapter dealt specifically with leadership at the local healthcare-system level, there are things about current healthcare systems processes at a broader level that also need to be examined and ideally changed. By "local healthcare system," we refer to the networks of hospitals and clinics that work closely together, sharing patients, and providing healthcare services. From a patient perspective, it's sort of like insurance coverage being in or out of network. The network, in this example, often coincides with the local healthcare system preferred by the insurance company, or in some cases the group of local healthcare systems within the network.

Solution #10 in this chapter is focuses on specific changes that need to be enacted at the broadest level of the healthcare system. Some of these changes may be initiated or at least advocated by local healthcare system leaders, but they often require support from politicians and government leaders in order to occur. We will discuss the current business model for most broad or national healthcare systems (Hennig-Schmidt et al., 2011), discuss one alternative that is emerging in the United States, and review broad recommendations by a panel of physician leaders, with a critical eye to the feasibility of their suggestions. Our hope is to identify a set of possible changes that may provide a workable and effective solution to burnout at the broad healthcare system level.

The Current Business Model

The current business model for most healthcare systems in which most physicians work is a fee-for-service model (Green, 2014). Particularly in the United States, physicians get paid by seeing patients, prescribing medications and procedures, and billing both the patient and their insurance company. Although other models exist in other countries (and this will be addressed in Chapter 15), the fee-for-service model remains the most prominent model for compensating physicians and others in the healthcare systems of the United States. As a consequence of the model, physician compensation, and to some extent the compensation of other healthcare personnel, depends primarily on volume. That is, the more patients you see and prescribe procedures and medications for, the more money that comes into the system to pay for all the things needed to maintain the system, including overhead (e.g., building space, utilities) and salaries.

An unintended consequence, a trickle-down effect, of the prevalent fee-for-service model is the exacerbation of some of the individual-level, team-level, and local system–level work issues that are known to cause burnout. As a prominent example, physician workload and workflow issues are widely accepted as a major source of burnout. Under the prevailing business model, doctors feel obligated to see more and more patients, thereby giving patients less and less of their time, while also expecting to provide high-quality services and desirable outcomes for the patient. After all, in a fee-for-service model, more patients means more money. We know that balancing those demands at the individual and team level may be problematic (see Chapters 6–10), particularly if the system itself does not provide a mechanism for opting out of the fee-for-service, piece-rate system. Patients can quickly become widgets on the conveyer belt within the metaphorical healthcare factory, with physicians essentially becoming critical-thinking line workers. The more satisfied, healthier-than-when-they-arrived widgets they can produce, the more financial resources enter the system for their benefit. The cap on the potential for salary for the entire system is set by the maximum number of patients the healthcare provider can manage to see. That is the situation as expressed over and over to John and Joe in their interviews and conversations with healthcare workers.

As a sidebar, note that we identify the prevailing volume-based compensation system as a form of piece-rate pay. In the past, workers in many industries were paid to some extent based on the number of units of product they produced. Commission-based compensation for sales representatives is a still-common current example. One of the obvious limitations of such a compensation system is that it puts pressure on the worker to do more and do it faster, in order to earn more. That pressure obviously can increase the risks of burnout. A second limitation of the piece-rate system is that, because it rewards production only, other desirable behaviors, including those related to teamwork, are unlikely to occur. As a personal example, John consulted with a clothing manufacturing company that had historically paid its production employees for the most part on a piece-rate system. Sew more sweatshirts and sweatpants, and get paid more. The company was inspired to introduce some of the critical elements of a high-performance organization, and wanted to encourage some of their senior employees to serve as "shift captains," coaching and training junior employees. Leaders in the company were initially disappointed that candidates for the captain role were reluctant to take it on. But the reasons were obvious. It was only when the pay system was adjusted to reward (not punish) time away from the sewing machine that the captain system worked.

The predominant fee-for-service model in itself imposes some level of burnout risk on healthcare providers, regardless of the individual or team-based mitigation strategies they may implement. A solution at the broad systems level would involve to some extent disentangling physician compensation from the volume-based, fee-for-service model. But how to change the monetary reward system to no longer require physicians to see twenty or more (sometimes many more) patients per clinic session? Additionally, some systems have quotas that are to be met, often labeled as "goals," but that are essentially numbers of patients to be seen per clinic hour or session. Setting goals or quotas is not an alternative to the fee-for-service model as it continues to apply the same pressure associated with the reward structure (i.e., meet the goal, keep the pay/job, and everyone's happy, right?). Instead, one recommendation that is beginning to gain visibility is to make compensation tied to patient satisfaction and outcomes (a so-called quality or value-based system), though the implementation of such systems has challenges and limitations of its own, and fee-for-service remains dominant.

We will next explore another option, one that is gaining traction especially among primary care physicians as a possible alternative to the piece-rate/fee-for-service system that is currently contributing in a major way to burnout among physicians. It should be noted that any changes to the compensation system will have both intended and unintended consequences, and a one-size-fits-all approach is usually not advisable (Mehta, 2015).

Concierge Medical Practice

A main alternative to volume-based compensation that is getting a lot of attention in the medical literature in the United States is so-called concierge medical practice. In such practices, the physician limits the number of patients in their practice and offers them more or less exclusive on-demand services for an annual fee. Instead of twenty or more patients per day, the physician may see eight to ten patients, but receive the same (or more) compensation, factoring in the annual fee. The advantages to the physician are clear and immediate. Burnout risk typically is greatly reduced or even eliminated, and financial freedom emerges without a feeling of inadequacy in responding to all the needs of patients. The advantage to patients includes longer, more in-depth visits with their primary care physician, shorter wait times, and the reality of being able to see the doctor the same or next day when emergencies arise. Additionally, and critically, an advantage to both doctor and patient is a greatly reduced chance of medical error. Overall, the patient and physician have a closer, more personal relationship than with the prevailing volume-based model.

The concierge medical practice may sound like a dream come true, and it is a model embraced by growing numbers of primary care physicians. As beneficial as the model is to the physician and their patients, there are limitations and unintended consequences. A major limitation is that such a system may work only with primary care physicians. Other medical practitioners, such as specialists, may not be able to implement such a model. It doesn't fit the realities of their practice. That being said, the primary care physician is often the first point of contact for the patient, and better clinical outcomes by this "first gatekeeper" reduce the likelihood of passing error on to specialists, pharmacists, and others in the chain of healthcare providers.

As an example of an unintended consequence, who is most likely to be able to afford the out-of-pocket expense of even a very modest yearly fee? Likely those who are generally well off financially. Thus, primary care physicians working within the concierge model will likely see a less diverse patient group, and it is possible that the lines and demands on the open clinics will increase. Not surprisingly, low socioeconomic and minority individuals are on average likely to suffer more under these systems. In other words, as we help to solve one major problem – physician burnout – we may create or at least add to another, namely, restricted access to primary medical care for some demographics. A two-tiered system might eventually emerge, creating further social disparity. That all being said, the self-report assessments of primary care physicians who adopt a concierge approach are extremely positive, and "workarounds" have been developed to minimize problems, including the unequal-access issue identified above. Some of the concierge models support doctors in taking on some of their less advantaged patients on a pro bono basis, still without overburdening their practice or significantly reducing their compensation.

Considerations from the National Commission on Physician Payment Reform

Given the well-documented limitations of the fee-for-service model, and some of the concerns about and potential limitations of the concierge alternative, it is important to consider how to change systems in ways that obtain the benefits of the concierge approach while avoiding or minimizing the consequence of restricted access. The solution may well follow some of the broad recommendations originating from the National Commission on Physician Payment Reform (Siddiqui et al., 2014). This body made several suggestions with the goal to maximize clinical outcomes, enhance patient and physician satisfaction and autonomy, and provide cost-effective care. We share their relevant suggestions here and discuss them in relation to the potential impact on the healthcare system and physician burnout. Note that the suggestions as stated are broad, aspirational goals. Little if any implementation detail is provided.

1. *Payers of healthcare, including both patients and insurance companies, should endeavor to eliminate stand-alone fee-for-service payment to medical practices.* Given the limitations, inherent inefficiencies, and potentially unethical financial incentives, it is no surprise that the first and perhaps most challenging recommendation is, simply and bluntly, to end the fee-for-service model. Many of the subsequent recommendations/suggestions center on how this critical and fundamental change might be accomplished. Any effective new alternative system would surely involve reduced workload and improved workflow, thereby greatly benefiting physicians from a burnout perspective

2. *New models of care that focus on quality and value should be tested over a five-year period before incorporating them into practice.* As scientists who prefer to test hypotheses *before* concluding that something should be done in practice, and indeed to pilot a research study before conducting it in full, this recommendation makes quite a bit of sense to us. From a practical perspective, though, it may be hard to justify such a long delay between testing and implementation. Thus, we recommend a middle ground that does not ignore the need for testing, but does not delay action for so long. We recommend a pilot approach that would involve initiating new models immediately in a subset of systems and tracking the data from day one. If, after a year, the early indicators are positive and consequences (intended or otherwise) are satisfactory, then consider expanding the model into more systems/

areas within systems. Repeat that constant evaluation process over time so that in five years, the new model is potentially completely in place; if it is not an improvement, it has already been dismissed, and another option is being tested. After all, the burnout problem is not just going to go away during this time unless action is taken, by both leaders and workers. We emphasize that such a pilot-study approach, while having the advantage of speed of implementation and ongoing testing of effectiveness, must be monitored carefully. There may well be challenges if very different systems of compensation and other incentives exist side by side. We have seen examples of pilot programs in manufacturing settings where teams working on a new automated production line, with different job descriptions and a different pay and bonus structure, failed, largely because of internal frictions with other shifts or departments that were not on the new system. This is not an insurmountable problem, but it must be monitored.

3. *Recalibrate the fee-for-service payment system immediately given that it will remain the system for some time.* Reasonably so, this suggestion recognizes that the shift away from fee-for-service will not occur overnight. The implement-test-assess process just suggested will take time, perhaps five years, perhaps longer, and given that government-based insurance is common among older adults and low-income families and follows the fee-for-service approach, the suggestion here is a pragmatic one indeed. That is, we know there are problems with the fee-for-service system relative to how much a physician is reimbursed for various procedures. Adjusting those to reflect reality and making changes in care plan/practice is essential to continuing care during the transition, whatever form that transition takes. As with the other recommendations, no specific guidelines are offered as to just what adjustments or recalibrations should ideally be made, and how physician compensation would be affected.

4. *Insurance providers use codes in a complex system to determine how much they pay for procedures, and these need to be evaluated and adjusted more frequently to keep pace with medical innovation.* In the United States, both Medicare and private insurers rely on lists of codes for pricing payment for medical procedures. In time those codes become outdated. Costs for procedures tend to go down over time. Locations where procedures occur, in- versus out-patient, greatly impact the costs. When these codes are not updated there can be artificial incentives for physicians and the healthcare system to prescribe procedures that may or may not be efficient or necessary. Constant or at

least frequent updates to these documents will help ensure accuracy in care. Again, this is essentially a stop-gap measure while the alternative payment models, with specifics yet to be determined, are tested and then implemented.

5. *New payment mechanisms need to be more transparent than current fee-for-service models and reimbursement should be equal for equivalent services.* Based on recent conversations with physicians, Joe learned that compensation is simply not a clear and transparent process for medical providers. This problem is due in part to the complexity of the multitude of insurers, government agencies, and others involved in determining reimbursement levels. However, part of the problem also is a lack of transparency on the part of healthcare systems concerning workload minimums, goals, and quotas. Achieving these minimums, goals, or quotas for numbers of patients seen does not consider the complexity of the patient need, the demand (or lack of demand) for the physician's specialty area, or other critical variables. From a burnout perspective, the ambiguity that all these things create only exacerbates the issue for the physician. Hence the broad recommendation to clarify, be transparent, and pay equally for equivalent work makes a great deal of sense.

6. *As fee-for-service remains for some time, new contracts using this model must include both outcome-based performance and quality of care for reimbursement to proceed.* In other words, patient outcomes and patients' feelings about the service they receive should be part of the equation in determining the compensation for services rendered. The growing pressure toward focusing more directly on patient outcomes and patient satisfaction, touched on earlier, will most likely require physicians to see fewer patients so as to ensure that needs are met, thus, at minimum, slowing down the conveyer belt in the factory of healthcare (Halbesleben & Rathert, 2008; Panagioti et al., 2018). Although this is *not* the single best or only solution to the fee-for-service problem, it is something that would begin to give breathing room for the new models to be tested and for more permanent, long-term solutions to be identified. Further, there is another important reason for caution in implementing a focus on patient outcome and satisfaction for compensation strategies. Studies showed that nearly a third of physicians in emergency care were considering leaving the job or even the profession if patient satisfaction was the main or only driver of compensation (Zgierska et al., 2014). While there may be any of a number of reasons that physicians would react in this way,

clearly the answer is more complicated than a complete switch to some quality-based metric for compensation.

7. *Telemedicine became much more readily used due to the pandemic, and the fee-for-services reimbursement methods should reflect this change and encourage the use of virtual tools to ensure care for the broadest reach of patients.* Primarily among smaller practices, telemedicine was becoming common pre-pandemic. For context, in 2019, approximately 22 percent of physicians used telehealth; this number spiked to 80 percent of physicians in 2020 (Drees, 2020). However, fee-for-service models were not well equipped to reimburse these services properly, though they tended to enhance care in terms of increasing frequency of check-ups with physicians, responsiveness of patient needs, and overall patient satisfaction (Hailey et al., 2002). For example, in rural areas where seeing the physician in person may require many hours of travel by car, telemedicine has been providing potentially life-saving care in a timelier manner. With the pandemic came a huge push to use telemedicine in general, and now payment systems have been required to catch up and to maintain transparency in reimbursement for telemedicine. The pandemic accelerated both the adoption of telemedicine processes and the figuring out of how to appropriately charge for remote services (PYA, 2020).

8. *In considering alternatives to the fee-for-service system, healthcare systems should look for fixed payment systems that could provide additional cost savings and better quality.* In other words, when looking at potential system alternatives (for a few options, see Calsyn and Lee, 2012), targeting ways to significantly reduce costs and improve the quality of care should be part of the equation. This is the National Commission's way of reminding healthcare system leaders and workers to be mindful of the consequences of the new systems of compensation that are currently available or that could be designed and built. The decision makers are reminded to not allow the promise of a new system to outweigh the aims of reducing cost for patients and providing quality care. The hope is that these potentially competing goals can harmonize.

It should be noted that some of these strategic changes are completely or largely within the power of the leaders of local healthcare systems, while others may require a professional society, community, or nation-level effort. Ultimately, the implementation of this solution will require collaboration across levels within the local system and including the broader national healthcare system.

Summing Up

In sum, solution #10 is really about changing the current business model in our healthcare systems to better reflect the espoused values of the physicians, creating a compensation structure that is based on meaningful metrics other than the number of patients seen. Most generally, our hope is that healthcare systems will be willing to deal head-on with the potential crisis of care amid the actual crisis of burnout. As demand continues to increase, the pipeline for new physicians will also need to be addressed, which again is part of the changes needed at the national level of healthcare, in most countries. While we have not dealt directly with this issue, there are physician shortages in many parts of the United States and other countries, and there is no indication that medical school enrollments are up to the point of addressing those shortages (Zhang et al., 2020).

The COVID-19 Effect

The coronavirus pandemic necessitated a monumental change in how healthcare is delivered. Specifically, telehealth visits increased by 154 percent in March 2020, and that increase has maintained and in some areas continued to rise through the pandemic (Koonin et al., 2020). Physicians were suddenly required to provide as much care as they could possibly give in a virtual environment. At the same time, healthcare systems, insurance companies, and government medical laws had to adjust to figure out how to best compensate healthcare providers in this not totally new, but suddenly ubiquitous healthcare delivery process. What this taught Joe and John is that change in the healthcare industry across nearly every system in the United States and United Kingdom can and does happen. However, our hope is that it won't take another pandemic or similar global event to provide an impetus to change healthcare systems at the broadest level to mitigate burnout.

Key Takeaways

- Changes in healthcare system processes are complex, difficult to enact, but possible.
- The current fee-for-service model for compensation creates a conveyor belt, factory-style environment for patients and physicians.
- Workload in the current fee-for-service system is not sustainable, so options (e.g., the concierge service model) need to be considered.

- The sudden changes required by COVID-19 relative to telemedicine and compensation for those services proves that changes in healthcare system processes do happen.

REFERENCES

Calsyn, M., & Lee, E. O. (2012). Alternatives to fee-for-service payments in health care. Center for American Progress. www.americanprogress.org/issues/healthcare/reports/2012/09/18/38320/alternatives-to-fee-for-service-payments-in-health-care/.

Drees, J. (2020, October 6). Physician telehealth usage increased 58% since 2019, survey finds. *Becker's Hospital Review.* www.beckershospitalreview.com/telehealth/physician-telehealth-usage-increased-58-since-2019-survey-finds.html.

Green, E. P. (2014). Payment systems in the healthcare industry: An experimental study of physician incentives. *Journal of Economic Behavior & Organization, 106*, 367–378.

Hailey, D., Roine, R., & Ohinmaa, A. (2002). Systematic review of evidence for the benefits of telemedicine. *Journal of Telemedicine and Telecare, 8* (Suppl. 1), 1–30. https://doi.org/10.1258/1357633021937604

Halbesleben, J. R., & Rathert, C. (2008). Linking physician burnout and patient outcomes: Exploring the dyadic relationship between physicians and patients. *Health Care Management Review, 33*(1), 29–39.

Hennig-Schmidt, H., Selten, R., & Wiesen, D. (2011). How payment systems affect physicians' provision behaviour: An experimental investigation. *Journal of Health Economics, 30*(4), 637–646.

Koonin, L. M., Hoots, B., Tsang, C. A., Leroy, Z., Farris, K., Jolly, B., . . . & Harris, A. M. (2020). Trends in the use of telehealth during the emergence of the COVID-19 pandemic – United States, January–March 2020. *Morbidity and Mortality Weekly Report, 69*(43), 1595.

Mehta, S. J. (2015). Patient satisfaction reporting and its implications for patient care. *AMA Journal of Ethics, 17*(7), 616–621.

Panagioti, M., Geraghty, K., Johnson, J., Zhou, A., Panagopoulou, E., Chew-Graham, C., . . . & Esmail, A. (2018). Association between physician burnout and patient safety, professionalism, and patient satisfaction: A systematic review and meta-analysis. *JAMA Internal Medicine, 178*(10), 1317–1331.

PYA. (2020, April 20). COVID-19 quick hit: Telehealth compensation. www.pyapc.com/insights/telehealth-compensation-covid-19/.

Siddiqui, M., Joy, S., Elwell, D., & Anderson, G. F. (2014). The National Commission on Physician Payment Reform: Recalibrating fee-for-service and transitioning to fixed payment models. *Journal of General Internal Medicine, 29*(5), 700–702.

Zgierska, A., Rabago, D., & Miller, M. M. (2014). Impact of patient satisfaction ratings on physicians and clinical care. *Patient Preference and Adherence, 8,* 437–446. https://doi.org/10.2147/PPA.S59077.

Zhang, X., Lin, D., Pforsich, H., & Lin, V. W. (2020). Physician workforce in the United States of America: Forecasting nationwide shortages. *Human Resources for Health, 18*(1), 8. https://doi.org/10.1186/s12960-020-0448-3

CHAPTER 15

Solution #11: Make Changes in National Healthcare

In our day-to-day, we don't have time to talk about "national healthcare," but something's got to give!
—Internal medicine physician

The final potential solution is likely outside the direct influence of most individuals who might read this. That's because our proposed final solution relies on national healthcare regulations, policies, and laws being changed or substantially adjusted in favor of reducing the burnout crisis for physicians, nurses, and other healthcare providers. Further, these broadest system-level efforts would also change the experience for patients for the better, much better. However, change of the magnitude we envision is not usually fully embraced, easy to enact, or likely to occur without substantial help from multiple directions. Stakeholders at all levels must do their part to act to create change, rather than be acted on by change. We encourage those with an active interest in healthcare (and that should include all of us) to engage in the process, lobby, vote, encourage leaders, become a leader, write letters, and be involved in every way possible so that major change becomes possible. Hopefully, together, with enough pushing by physicians, healthcare system leaders, patients, and any other stakeholders, we can make our healthcare systems better at the national level.

It is important to recognize the different kinds of healthcare systems at the national level across countries. In each of these cases, there is detailed regulation and thorough involvement of the government in dictating how healthcare delivery is supposed to operate. We will explore four of the primary options. Each of these possible national systems has some pros and cons, some intended and some unintended consequences. Let's examine and assess the options.

We will start with a hypothetical system that, while a logical possibility, with parallels in other aspects of national economies, is not applied per se in any existing healthcare system.

The Free-Market Medical System

The free-market healthcare system is a hypothetical system of healthcare where prices for healthcare goods and services would be freely set by agreements between healthcare providers and patients (Testa & Block, 2013). Under these conditions, the basic principles of supply and demand would be allowed to operate without regulation from government, or with bare minimum governmental intervention. Those in favor of a free-market healthcare system argue that healthcare systems that rely on insurance or substantial government involvement result in higher costs and widespread inefficiencies, including longer lines for care, among others. Skeptics of the free-market approach assert that healthcare in an unregulated environment would lead to both unfair and inefficient outcomes, such that poorer individuals might be unable to afford care altogether.

In a free-market healthcare system, control of the workload and workflow might well be more under the control of the physician, potentially reducing burnout. However, if the fee-for-service business model still prevailed, it is unlikely that physicians would voluntarily reduce their workload (and their pay). Thus, it is unclear if the control that could emerge in a free-market healthcare system would offset the free-market forces that would still pressure physicians to do more and more. Further, and critically, no country appears to have a free-market healthcare system, so it is hard to draw any definitive conclusions about the potential consequences, intended and otherwise, of such a system over time.

The US economy is largely a free-market system, and yet the medical enterprise has not at all embraced that approach. One critical implication of a free-market healthcare system, namely, that some people would have access to care (those that could afford it) while others would not, seems to be a central reason that the United States has not embraced the free-market healthcare model (Testa & Block, 2013). Regardless, we can only speculate what such a model would look like at this point, as no country on the planet has a fully free-market healthcare system.

The Socialized Medicine System

The socialized medicine healthcare system is a system in which the government provides for the healthcare of its citizens in all respects (Neeman, 2019). In systems of this nature, the government regulates, runs, and controls all healthcare facilities and associated providers. Healthcare services in a socialized medicine system are funded by taxes, with taxpayers usually paying a much higher tax rate when compared to taxpayers in other countries without socialized medicine. However, in return for the higher tax rate, citizens receive "free" health services and low-cost medicines.

Proponents of socialized medicine (and there are many) argue that such a system creates greater equity for all citizens. It should also save lives because more people have healthcare, since it is provided to all citizens of the nation. Proponents also argue that because healthcare is embedded in the governmental system, public health and welfare initiatives are more supported; there is greater overall productivity among the citizenry; and, overall, money is saved (Neeman, 2019). It must be noted that all these claims are generally supported with the exception of the productivity of the citizenry, arguably due to other associated economic pressures outside the socialized health system paradigm (Slaybaugh, 2019). It is hoped and expected that citizens in a socialized medicine system will be more compliant with public health initiatives and also more mindful of the importance of regular maintenance of their own health. Unfortunately, this tenet of socialized medicine has apparently not been fulfilled in practice.

Critics of socialized medicine point to countries (e.g., Germany, Israel, Norway, Japan, and Austria, to name a few) that have implemented this system and note long wait times for services, some rationing of care, and much higher taxes (Neeman, 2019). Additionally, critics point out the obvious fact that socialized medicine eliminates competition, which is a major driver for innovation and quality of care (Ubel, 2019). Without competition for patients and compensation, what is the motivation for identifying new and more efficient ways of conducting procedures? These and other concerns (especially the long lines for medical procedures and rationing of care) are commonly and passionately raised by critics of socialized medicine.

Our view is that the proponents and critics are both correct. Yes, more people have access to care, and yes, there are long lines and rationing. From the critical perspective of physician burnout, it is unlikely that a sudden increase in patients' access to care would benefit them in terms of demand on their time. In fact, under these conditions, the already strapped healthcare providers would most likely be inundated with new patients, and doctors would likely feel obligated to try to do more, if anything exacerbating the burnout issue. Thus, socialized medicine may also not be the right answer for physician burnout, particularly given that reported levels of burnout are still very high in countries that have this system (Locke, 2019).

The Hybrid System

The hybrid healthcare system has some elements of both the free market and socialized medicine in hopes of getting the best of both systems (Ridic et al., 2012). The United States uses this approach to healthcare with both a relatively free-market insurance-based system and Medicaid/Medicare for financially disadvantaged families and older adults. Regulation in the United States in the hybrid system has enabled and constrained healthcare in interesting ways, generally exacerbating rather than mitigating burnout among physicians and other healthcare providers. Obviously, the proponents of the hybrid model argue that the system has the best attributes of both free-market and socialized medicine. The detractors argue that it also has the worst elements of both systems. The answer, we think, is they are once again both correct.

From a physician burnout perspective, the hybrid system is the source of most of the hard data and anecdotal stories that are shared in this volume. In other words, the hybrid model, which is what is seen in the United States, has yielded a vast amount of evidence as to what not to do in terms of burnout. Thus, we obviously could not recommend simply maintaining this system as it currently stands as a means of reducing burnout among physicians and other providers.

The Universal Healthcare System

In recent years there has been a groundswell of interest in the idea of a universal healthcare system. The universal healthcare system is a system that ideally provides high-quality medical services to all citizens (Amadeo, 2020). Socialized medicine bears some similarity to universal healthcare, but universal healthcare is the broader, more inclusive term and requires separate attention here. Once again, in most universal healthcare systems seen around the world (e.g., the United Kingdom, Poland, Sweden, and Denmark), the government provides healthcare to all citizens regardless of the ability to pay into the system. Those funds often come from taxes, like what one would see in Canada (Ridic et al., 2012). A unique feature of universal healthcare ideology that is less present or at least less emphasized in socialized medicine is the focus on high quality of care and the implementation of strategies such as national healthcare grants for research that specifically incentivize innovation and continuous improvement (Amadeo, 2020; Ridic et al., 2012).

The advantages of such a system, enacted with quality in mind, are the possibilities of lower overall healthcare costs, reduced administrative costs, enhanced equality of care (i.e., available to everyone), and standard practice across hospitals/clinics. Proponents of universal healthcare assert that such a system likely would promote public health practices (e.g., masking behavior commonly required during the coronavirus pandemic; Amadeo, 2020). Still others argue that universal healthcare would lead to a healthier public because the government would more fully require early childhood preventive care, such as vaccinations (Amadeo, 2020).

Disadvantages, to some degree, mirror those of socialized medicine. For example, some would argue that universal healthcare in all its iterations would create long wait times and rationing of procedures. For example, in the United Kingdom, 41 percent of patients wait a month or more to receive care (World Population Review, 2021). Additionally, under most such systems, healthy people are paying for those who are sick through the tax system, and there is less incentive to stay healthy as there are no immediately incurred costs for seeing the doctor. Alternatively, because doctor visits are perceived as free, more people participate in healthcare and may therefore engage in more healthy behaviors. Further, universal systems mean that governments' budgets would swell dramatically, and control and choice of care might be impacted by government regulators more than by patient needs and requests. Perhaps most problematic for the US citizenry may be that universal healthcare would mean more involvement of the government in healthcare decisions, reducing or removing personal choice in care processes and providers.

Once again, the improvements in burnout are still slow to occur under most universal healthcare options, at least initially. We know from research that people who see the doctor for regular wellness visits and physicals do tend to be healthier over time. Thus, even though we agree that the initial demand on the system would be dramatic, if care was provided and preventive behavior became normalized, then the long-term drain on the physicians could be reduced. However, getting to that point would likely burn out most of the healthcare providers along the way.

Regulation within the Hybrid US Healthcare System

Although the examples relevant to burnout that are provided in our book are predominantly from the United States, healthcare regulations in the United Kingdom and many other countries are creating or contributing to the burnout crisis as well (De Hert, 2020). Burnout among physicians is a global issue, not limited to any country or any particular healthcare system, as clearly articulated in earlier chapters.

There are two major areas of healthcare regulation and government involvement in the United States that, as they currently stand, contribute substantially to physician burnout and are in urgent need of revision. First, governmental statutes related to electronic health records requirements inadvertently create an environment that contributes in a major way to burnout among physicians. In 2009, the Obama administration introduced an electronic health records mandate, with the requirement that physicians had to show meaningful use of digital medical records by 2014 or see their Medicare and Medicaid payments reduced. Thus, healthcare systems and physicians not wanting to see their pay and bottom lines reduced, swiftly implemented EHR, requiring physicians themselves to enter information into these systems. The intended consequence was to make available any person's medical records to their care provider at a moment's notice, which of course would be vital in an emergency.

As previously stated in Chapter 12, one unintended consequence of the implementation of EHR is that physicians and other healthcare providers now log many hours entering information into EHR, often after hours, in the evenings, on weekends, and during holidays. In fact, just about any healthcare institution can see when their people are logged into EHR. While consulting with several hospitals across the country, we helped identify spikes in EHR work occurring after hours and noted a particularly problematic spike at 9 p.m. on Sunday evenings. Given the impact of work-family spillover and excessive job demands on burnout, US government regulators need to consider alternatives or adjustments to the EHR requirements so that the positive intended consequences remain while the negative unintended consequences do not inadvertently fuel the burnout crisis (Arndt et al., 2017; Robinson & Kersey, 2018; Tajirian et al., 2020).

Second, Medicare and Medicaid cover more than 128 million Americans and impose enormous regulatory burdens on physicians and the healthcare system in general, while paying considerably less than private insurance companies. This difference is so stark that in many cases, the government payment does not even cover the cost of providing care to the beneficiaries. This has led to many healthcare providers limiting the number of Medicaid and Medicare patients they will see, further augmenting the burden of care on certain areas of the healthcare system that are often ill-equipped for the increase in patient demand.

Again, although these are US-based examples, the broader implications are clear: Government regulations in general have the potential to exacerbate or even create the burnout crisis. However, governments can also adjust, change, or put new regulations in place to directly address and help mitigate physician burnout. Echoing the recommendations made by the panel of healthcare CEOs in 2016, covered in Chapter 13, we suggest that physicians, nurses, other healthcare providers, and healthcare systems leaders take proactive steps to get involved with their government representatives as well as with professional organizations (e.g., the AMA) to encourage change via legislation and other legal means. We recognize that these efforts may require years of attention and consistent messaging. Thus, organizational leaders have an ongoing responsibility to incorporate proactive communication to government leaders and legislators with responsibility for oversight of the healthcare systems.

Barriers to Proposed Solutions

Our proposed solution at the broad systems level is to significantly adjust the national healthcare systems, including the laws and regulations that support them, to allow for a more humane, lower-stress work environment for physicians and other healthcare workers. However, as the review of current systems shows, that's not as easy as it might have sounded, even when we said it was probably a bigger challenge than any one reader of our book would be able to tackle in a lifetime. The major barrier for solution #11 in the United States is convincing lawmakers to work to change entitlement programs like Medicaid and Medicare as well as other aspects of the current system such as the role of major insurance companies. Doing so, even with the intended consequence of adequately compensating physicians and providing funds for much-needed services for beneficiaries, will prove challenging. Still, there are many across the political spectrum who would be in favor of these changes as they would assist in alleviating physician burnout and also improve patient well-being, reduce suffering, and enhance quality of life for healthcare workers and their patients.

Summing Up

In sum, healthcare systems are complex systems embedded within the culture and environment of the countries where they operate. Free-market, socialized, hybrid, and universal healthcare systems all have their pros and cons, their opportunities and challenges. However, none of them appears to create and support an environment that adequately addresses the issue of burnout among physicians. In short, adoption or continuation of any existing system as currently implemented will not solve the problem.

Rather, healthcare leaders and government officials must consider alternatives to the systems that exist, enact laws and provisions to address the burnout issue, and collaboratively evolve their healthcare systems into more effective ones.

The COVID-19 Effect

Although admittedly an opinion article, Maizland and Felter (2020) compared six countries and their healthcare systems during the early phase of the pandemic. Essentially, they asked the question, "How was the initial and ongoing response to the pandemic different in these countries?" They concluded the following:

- Taiwan had an effective coronavirus response.
- The United Kingdom had a delayed effort.
- South Korea had a very swift response.
- Australia avoided widespread outbreak entirely.
- The Netherlands had a partial lockdown.
- The United States had a disjointed response.

At least from this article, one might conclude the universal health care system in Taiwan is the way to go in a pandemic. However, such a conclusion would ignore the complex cultural environment in Taiwan, including the largely collectivistic culture and subsequent widespread compliance with a "what is good for the group is good for me" attitude. In the end, our conclusion is that, on the issue of which system is good for burnout, the answer is far more complex than simply one system over another.

Key Takeaways

- There are several different healthcare systems currently enacted in countries all over the world, and none of them seems to be immune to the burnout issue.
- When considering which healthcare system is best for a given country, one must consider culture, environment, and unique government regulations of each country.
- A more realistic and effective solution relative to healthcare systems is an adjustment approach, where leaders of organizations and leaders in government look for ways to change laws and regulations to target burnout-related issues, and then implement and monitor those changes.

REFERENCES

Amadeo, K. (2020, March 13). Why America Is the only rich country without universal health care. The Balance. www.thebalance.com/universal-health-care-4156211.

Arndt, B. G., Beasley, J. W., Watkinson, M. D., Temte, J. L., Tuan, W. J., Sinsky, C. A., & Gilchrist, V. J. (2017). Tethered to the EHR: Primary care physician workload assessment using EHR event log data and time-motion observations. *The Annals of Family Medicine, 15*(5), 419–426.

De Hert S. (2020). Burnout in healthcare workers: Prevalence, impact and preventative strategies. *Local and Regional Anesthesia, 13,* 171–183. https://doi.org/10.2147/LRA.S240564.

Locke, T. (2019). Medscape global physicians' burnout and lifestyle comparisons. Medscape. www.medscape.com/slideshow/2019-global-burnout-comparison-6011180#4.

Maizland, L., & Felter, C. (2020). Comparing six health-care systems in a pandemic. Council on Foreign Relations.org. www.cfr.org/backgrounder/comparing-six-health-care-systems-pandemic.

Neeman, E. (2019, February 26). What is socialized medicine? Everything you need to know. First Quote Health. www.firstquotehealth.com/health-insurance-news/what-is-socialized-medicine#:~:text=The%20Pros%20And%20Cons%20Of%20Socialized%20Medicine&text=It%20makes%20healthcare%20more%20accessible,elimination%20of%20competition%20in%20healthcare.

Ridic, G., Gleason, S., & Ridic, O. (2012). Comparisons of health care systems in the United States, Germany and Canada. *Materia Socio-Medica, 24*(2), 112–120. https://doi.org/10.5455/msm.2012.24.112-120.

Robinson, K. E., & Kersey, J. A. (2018). Novel electronic health record (EHR) education intervention in large healthcare organization improves quality, efficiency, time, and impact on burnout. *Medicine, 97*(38).

Slaybaugh, C. (2019, July 2). International healthcare systems: The US versus the world. Axene Health Partners,. https://axenehp.com/international-healthcare-systems-us-versus-world/.

Tajirian, T., Stergiopoulos, V., Strudwick, G., Sequeira, L., Sanches, M., Kemp, J., ... & Jankowicz, D. (2020). The influence of electronic health record use on physician burnout: Cross-sectional survey. *Journal of Medical Internet Research, 22*(7), e19274.

Testa, P., & Block, W. E. (2013). Applying the free market philosophy to healthcare. *Humanomics, 29*(2), 105–114.

Ubel, P. (2019, January 13). What socialized medicine would mean for your health. *Forbes.* www.forbes.com/sites/peterubel/2018/11/21/what-socialized-medicine-would-mean-for-your-health/?sh=fc4bc76e9a99.

World Population Review. (2021). Health care wait times by country 2021. Retrieved on September 22, 2021, from https://worldpopulationreview.com/country-rankings/health-care-wait-times-by-country.

CHAPTER 16

Saving the Burned-Out Physician

It's the unknown that is so scary ... not being able to see when and how the crisis will pass ... that's what's causing my stress.

—Lab technician

At the macro-societal level, we have to change the system. No eighty-hour weeks, less nonclinical administrative work for doctors. Fundamental changes in how medicine is practiced now. At the micro-personal level, take time off, reduce your load, spend time with the family (social support), exercise ... get clear on "what's important to me" ... change your approach, or get another job. At the team level, communicate and watch out for each other.

—Medical school professor

Our purpose in writing this book was to define the workplace syndrome of burnout in general, describe in some detail the experience of burnout among physicians and other medical workers, make the connection between burnout and medical error, identify where and why such errors occur, and provide a series of potential solutions for consideration by both medical professionals at all levels and those whom they are called on to serve on a daily basis, their patients.

Briefly recapping, burnout is the psychological and physical feeling of simply being used up and empty, exhausted at the end of a workday, work week, or work life in general. The profound physical and emotional fatigue is accompanied by cynicism and depersonalization, and feelings of low or no effectiveness. The common symptoms include psychological depression (a particularly prominent accompaniment to burnout), anxiety, fatigue, and cognitive and behavioral deficits as well as a wide range of physical symptoms associated with stress. Physicians and other healthcare providers are at particular risk for burnout, for reasons we have explored in depth. In general, their heavy workload and relatively low autonomy combine to add to the stress of their job. And stress that is prolonged and unmanaged at work is the culprit, the primary trigger for burnout.

A critically important and serious effect of burnout is greatly heightened risk of medical error, and it must be noted that knowledge that an error has been committed adds greatly to the stress of the physician or other healthcare worker (the so-called second victim effect). As burnout is widely identified as a crisis in healthcare, so is the magnitude of medical error, including avoidable fatal errors. The estimates are staggering, even by the most conservative estimates. Critical errors of many types can occur at any step in the extended process of healthcare-services delivery, most critically in initial diagnosis and treatment. Such errors have root causes in individual factors, teamwork factors, and overall systems factors, as we have identified in this book.

The medical burnout crisis is by no means limited to the United States. Our brief overview of the issue outside the United States, especially in the United Kingdom but also in other Western and non-Western countries, finds the same issues. The data from all sources are closely similar. And while burnout in practicing physicians is prominently studied, it is by no means limited to them, as we have repeatedly emphasized. Parallel research with nurses, physicians' assistants, medical students, and pharmacists (among others in the chain of healthcare delivery) points out the same issues. Indeed, as we reviewed the transcripts of our many interviews, we were struck by the fact that the central issues identified by our interviewees were so remarkably similar, whether the individual was a doctor or professor in a major medical school, a laboratory technician, a primary care physician, a medical student, or a pharmacist. While their day-to-day work differed, their experience with burnout and error was essentially the same. Indeed, with a very few minor edits, the full transcripts of our interviews would be virtually identical.

Thankfully, there are individual, team, management, organization, government, and professional society strategies that we propose as solutions, or at least potential solutions that can and should be implemented in order to address the crisis. These solutions are highly interdependent, as illustrated in Figure 16.1.

As depicted here, solutions that occur at broader, more encompassing national or local systems levels – that is, the outer rings in the figure – likely influence all levels identified by the inner rings. So, at the outermost level, broad governmental and professional society mandates and guidelines will necessarily influence policies and procedures at the local organizational level. Local hospital systems, clinics, and private practices must comply with governmental regulations, and additionally aim to follow best-practice strategies as identified by the American Medical Association

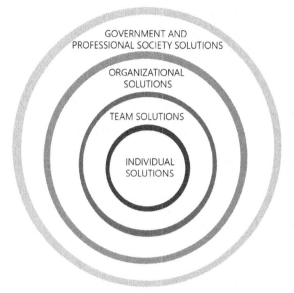

Figure 16.1   Interdependence of solutions.

and other professional societies. The local organization-level requirements and guidelines, set by hospitals, clinics, and other settings in which doctors and other providers operate, will set limits and establish policies and procedures that affect how teams can operate. And, in turn, team-level solutions, consistent with the advice and requirements of the government and professional society levels and of the organizational level, will impact individuals and their behavior. Thus, the most impactful, furthest-reaching changes would occur at the government and professional society levels, and the influence of those solutions would affect every inner circle in turn, as identified here. Effective solutions in the outer rings make it more likely that the inner rings will benefit and that solutions at those more local levels can work. By the same token, solutions in the outer rings that backfire have unintended negative consequences and in fact add stress to teams and individuals, making it more likely that individual doctors will suffer burnout, with the attendant increase in the likelihood of medical error.

Let's look at the rings of influence from the other direction. The individual healthcare provider is at the center. The effectiveness of those individuals depends on a number of factors, definitely including the effectiveness of the team in which they operate. Any team dysfunction will negatively impact their stress level and the quality of their work. The

effectiveness of the team is impacted by the local-system policies, procedures, and protocols of their organization. Their organization operates
within requirements set by broader-system regulatory/compliance requirements. Let's return to the individual level. Physicians, who are humans
with all the personal and family stresses we all deal with, have life-or-death
responsibility. They have heavy workloads and other requirements set by
their organizations. And more and more of their time is consumed by
administrative requirements set by their organizations and/or governmental regulations. All the pressures of the outer rings add to the pressures on
the individual. And the individual has the least direct influence over the
outer rings.

In some cases, a number of the systems-level solutions presented are
already in place, or at least are developing. Several of the physicians and
other medical professionals interviewed as part of the research for this book
described resiliency programs offered by their employers. In terms of
individual solutions as identified earlier, all of our interviewees identified
specific constructive efforts made by themselves and their families and
friends to help them cope with the stresses of their work and mitigate the
risk of burnout. The strategies they identified, especially social support and
self-care (exercise, diet, rest), are fully consistent with the recommendations in the individual stress-management literature, which help buffer the
individual from the risk of serious burnout. As a side note, none of our
interviewees self-reported any of the dysfunctional strategies that show up
so prominently in national survey data. Our interviewees also consistently
described how timely this topic is for them and for their families, in
general, but especially just now, as they manage working during the
pandemic and think about how they want the "next normal" to be.
Thus, as we introduced the "COVID-19 Effect" section across the chapters presented in this book, we identified ways in which the pandemic has
led to a sudden and dramatic spike in the stress level for all healthcare
providers, whether frontline or not; how that has increased the risk of
burnout and error; and, at the same time, how the pandemic has presented
an opportunity for individuals, teams, and healthcare systems to "hit the
reset button." Every crisis brings with it the opportunity, even the requirement, to rethink how we have been doing things, and to make constructive
change. So it is with the COVID-19 crisis. We believe that the role of the
physician and other healthcare providers will look different in the post-
pandemic era, though just how, we obviously can't completely predict.
Reflecting on the surge of stress and burnout risk that all have dealt with,
we do believe that better solutions will be identified and implemented at

all levels. They must. When the new pandemic crisis with its spike in burnout risk does pass, we can't just return to the old burnout crisis. If we are to continue to have new doctors in the pipeline, retain the ones we have, and reduce the extent of burnout and medical error, changes will have to be made.

This concluding chapter suggests three interrelated efforts that we hope our readers will want to undertake, and influence others to undertake, in order to turn around the current burnout crisis and help "save the burned out physician" and at the same time protect patients from burnout-related avoidable medical error. First, and of particular interest to the majority of readers, who are most likely physicians or other medical professionals, we provide a worksheet (Table 16.1) intended for reflection on your current situation and that of those around you within the healthcare system in which you operate. Second, we propose that all who read this book – medical professionals and other curious individuals (i.e., patients, caregivers, or just concerned citizens) – consider the "adaptive improvement model" (AIM) and fill in the self-assessment provided in Table 16.2. Third, we conclude with a brief discussion of the learning organization and the need for ongoing reflective processes such as the after-action review or debrief, both within the medical community and among individuals with their caregivers, and others. Our hope is that by encouraging you to deploy all three of these efforts, we may be able to save the burned-out physician by reducing their risk of burnout, improving the well-being of medical professionals, and saving lives from needless medical errors induced by known, fixable issues with our world medical system.

Summary of Solutions and Call for Reflection

To stem the tide of burnout, to save the burned-out physician, we provide here a brief summary list of the solutions, their general definitions (review Chapters 6–15 for more details), and a space for your reflection on each potential solution. The purpose here is to help you, the reader, reflect on where you are and how things stand in your workplace, for you as an individual (for physicians), for your team (medical professionals), for your organization and management (or the hospitals in which you might work), for your community. Concurrently, it is important to consider the approach currently being taken or not taken to implement these potential solutions.

We encourage you to use Table 16.1 and feel free to share it with your healthcare team, your management team, or any other stakeholders. The intent is to encourage you to begin to think about how these solutions are

Table 16.1. *Solutions and reflection notes*

	Potential solution	Broad definition	"Reflection notes"
Individual	1. Understand your personality	Interpret your characteristic patterns of thinking, feeling, and behaving	
	2. Take care of your physical self	Attend to the health aspects of your body, including diet, exercise, and sleep	
	3. Seek social support	Search for assistance from other individuals for emotional comfort	
	4. Follow the advice you would give patients	Act on the treatment recommendations you would give a patient in a similar situation as yourself	
Team	5. Effective team leadership	Leaders' positive ability to stimulate production while maintaining the trust and respect of the team	
	6. Collaborating team members	Individuals in a group who highlight team goals and actions in discussions and in their actions	
	7. Establishing and sustaining a positive team culture	Creating and maintaining an environment where team members approach individual responsibilities in a way that produces positive results for other members	
Management and organization	8. Changes in workflow in organizations	Differences in the sequence of work processes from initiation to completion	
	9. Changes in management practices for healthcare system leaders	Differences in the working methods used to improve work system effectiveness by those managing the healthcare systems	
	10. Changes in healthcare system process	Differences in the fee-for-service model that healthcare systems consider to assist with changing workload and physician/patient experiences	
Community/ Society	11. Changes in national healthcare	Differences in the organized provision of medical care to individuals and communities nationwide	

Table 16.2. *AIM worksheet*

CONTINUE
STOP
START

implemented, if at all, and to begin to consider specific approaches for their most effective implementation. As you engage in this reflective process, consider both how these solutions are or are not present in your environment/ situation as well as what might be done to change or improve on what exists.

The Adaptive Improvement Model (AIM)

Armed with your reflections in Table 16.1 based on the potential solutions provided, you are now prepared to consider the adaptive improvement model (AIM). AIM is meant to be applicable across levels, meaning that individuals, teams, managers, organizations, professional societies, and governments could essentially use the same approach in a collaborative way. AIM requires the consideration of three key ideas: things to continue doing, things to stop doing, and things to start doing. For ease of describing AIM, we focus on the individual level, but one could just as easily replace "I" with "we/us" (team) or even "our community" or "our hospital" (organization) or "our country."

Continue. In the AIM, "continue" refers to those things that are currently being done that one should keep doing. In essence, an individual should ask, "What am I doing in relation to my risk of burnout that I need to continue doing?" Answers could include social support, self-care (exercise, rest, diet), and any of the other healthy individual coping strategies identified and explained in earlier chapters. The key idea here is that most individuals (as well as, of course, teams, organizations, etc.) are doing some really good and appropriate things pertaining to stress management that helps stave off burnout and its consequences. We obviously mustn't abandon what is working to keep individuals healthy.

Stop. In the AIM, "stop" refers to those things that are being done that should be stopped immediately in order to mitigate burnout risk.

The individual should ask, "What am I doing in relation to my stress and burnout risk that I need to stop doing?" Answers might include the surprisingly common strategies of self-isolation, excessive drinking, or binge-eating, which were identified in Chapter 2. Answers might also include taking on new tasks, new patients, and new responsibilities when one is already maxed out in terms of workload. Again, the key idea here is that sometimes we engage in short-term survival tactics when we are dealing with a challenging situation, and those immediate go-to tactics (e.g., to heavily caffeinate to stave off sleep loss–related fatigue) are not healthy or sustainable. Furthermore, teams, organizations, and managers (and governments/societies) likely have things they need to stop doing.

Start. Start, in the AIM, refers to those things that individuals, teams, managers, organizations, and others need to start doing to begin to further stave off – in this case, burnout – and to mitigate undesirable outcomes, such as major errors. For example, an individual should ask, "What should I start doing to help me reduce my burnout?" If known positive strategies are not being implemented, answers could include engaging in self-care (Chapter 6), talking to a friend (Chapter 7), or reaching out to a team member (Chapters 9 and 10). Building on the reflection table just completed by you, your team, your manager, and other stakeholders, your set of things to start doing will reflect your own situation and will differ from that of others. Perhaps you identified a need to stop logging into EHR on Sunday evening, whereas others on your team may identify a need to take a regular lunch break, rather than taking a vending machine binge on the run. As you reflect on the things you've decided to start doing, consider the resources needed to make those solutions a reality. Hopefully, you've identified some "low hanging fruit" that will immediately provide relief and some additional capacity to tackle the harder things on your list.

Given these three elements of AIM, and having hopefully just completed some serious reflection on the provided solutions and your current situation, you are prepared (and perhaps your team with you) to complete the AIM worksheet provided in Table 16.2. Again, the goal is to complete each of the boxes, celebrating the things that you are doing well (continue), identifying the things that need to end (stop), and committing to the things that need to begin (start). As you do this, consider the various opportunities and barriers to success.

In fact, once you have collaboratively identified key things to start doing, there are likely a few questions that need to be answered. Using the specific example of starting a team training protocol for a healthcare team, Table 16.3 lists some of those potential questions and some prospective answers to them.

Table 16.3. *Team training example: Start logistical considerations*

Questions	Example answers for a training protocol
1. Who needs to be involved?	• All physicians, nurses, PAs, and others that comprise our team • Other folks in the organization interested in team development
2. What steps should be followed for carrying out this effort?	• Follow all internal procedures for introducing a new training • Perhaps emphasize the continuing medical education aspects of the training
3. When will the new initiative/effort begin?	• Set a date • Work with all key stakeholders to ensure broad participation
4. Where will implementation take place?	• Prepare for the physical or virtual logistics of the training • Identify conference room or other setting for the training • Consider the transfer of training options for broad implementation
5. How will the appropriate resources be identified, gathered, and used?	• Work with the team and administration to get the resources needed

Addressing such detailed questions will ensure that unforeseen barriers and opportunities for success are integrated into the plan for starting a new constructive effort. In reviewing these specific questions, note that, in general, even for individual-level activities, collaborative implementation by all affected parties is usually helpful, and often essential.

The Learning Organization and the Learning You

Building on the framework just discussed of engaging in reflection and taking AIM at priorities, we now turn our attention to some practical ways to think about how implementation of the evidence-based ideas presented in this book could help you move forward with burnout reduction and error-avoidance. First, consider the possibility of developing and implementing a sustainable "learning organization" within your workplace.

The concept of the learning organization is a relatively recent development in organizational theory, but it addresses a profoundly important issue that faces every organization. In simple terms, how does the organization gather information that helps it operate effectively, and how does it disseminate that information to teams and individuals who need it? That challenge is not handled well by many organizations. With a primary focus on "continuing to do what we do, but doing it better and better," there may be any of a number of developing threats and opportunities in the environment that are not seen by the internally focused organization. Also, some parts of the organization may be struggling with issues that other parts of the organization have already figured out how to handle. In our consulting roles, Joe and John have seen this issue repeatedly, where effective solutions have been developed and implemented in one part of the organization, but are unknown to other parts of the organization that are facing the same problems. True learning organizations have some mechanisms for scanning the external environment, to understand what is happening with technology, competitors, suppliers, customers, regulators, and so on that can impact how the organization does its business. Additionally, the learning organization must have mechanisms for scanning the internal environment and capturing internal knowledge as well. And all such knowledge must be made available to those who need it and must become part of the collective memory of the organization.

The logic of the learning organization is simple and straightforward and, frankly, not all that hard to implement. All that is required is to consider your workplace as a system (language that we have used throughout the book) embedded in a broader environment. While looking to improve internal functioning (continuing to do what we do well, but working to improve how we do it, stopping ineffective practices, and starting effective ones – i.e., AIM), also look at the relationship of your workplace with the broader environment in which it operates. Where are the threats that must be identified and addressed? Where are the opportunities that must be identified and capitalized on? How will we gather and disseminate the information, internal and external, that we need in order to respond adaptively to those inevitable challenges and opportunities?

The fundamental idea of the learning organization, as applied to healthcare, is simply to learn what effective solutions have been developed and implemented outside and inside your organization, and copy those best-practice ideas. Have others outside or inside your organization found better ways to reduce workload, to promote effective self-care strategies, to isolate and correct errors? If so, learn about and use those ideas.

Let's take some specific examples, with particular relevance to healthcare, namely, incident and close-call reporting, and "after-action reviews." In any system, including healthcare, documented incident reports are a major source of risk-assessment data. What kinds of incidents occur? Where and when do they happen? Looking for patterns as incidents are reviewed is a good starting point for risk assessment, an essential foundation for risk management. Learning organizations in all industries capture such data. As with other industries, healthcare systems should have such documented evidence. Such data, when captured and learned from, allow us to reduce error, to "keep that one from happening again." There is always the question, though, as to how accurate and complete such incident reports actually are. And as we noted earlier, that question of accuracy and completeness is particularly relevant in healthcare settings.

In addition to documenting adverse events, and in line with a team and individual learning approach, there is comparable value in capturing and learning from "close calls" in healthcare (which are more commonly called "near misses" in industrial settings). Data going back many decades support the general conclusion that close calls – also sometimes labeled "almost accidents" – are also a potentially rich source of data for identifying risk patterns and, therefore, for focusing mitigation strategies. In our work with HROs as well as other more traditional industries, Joe and John have encouraged companies to establish and use near-miss reporting and review systems. The viability of such systems depends critically on the level of trust that prevails in the organization in question, which in turn is strongly impacted by the consequences that follow a near-miss "confession." Furthermore, close-call reporting systems are now becoming more common in healthcare systems. For example, at Johns Hopkins medical system, the Patient Safety Net system receives more than 1,000 reports each month, with more than 90 percent of those reports representing close calls (Wu & Marks, 2013). Still, as with actual accident reporting, there is always the question of accuracy and completeness. And there is also the question of how the data are discussed and used.

Organizations that encourage and support near-miss conversations without exposing the individual in question to jeopardy are positioned to accurately identify their high-risk situations and develop and implement offset strategies to reduce the chance of the near miss turning into an accident at some point. In our experience there are sensitive "moment of truth" situations in which an individual talks about their error that resulted in a near miss. If leaders make it safe for their staff to do so, the organization gets better at risk identification and error reduction. If there is stigma and possible disciplinary action associated with such a conversation, such a conversation will not occur. Clearly, there are limits, but in general, an organization that accepts the reality that people make mistakes and learns from them rather than automatically punishing people for them will be a safer organization. As a side note, John has had the experience of encouraging several client companies to institute near-miss capturing systems. The long-term benefits are obvious. But a common outcome is that at first there are a lot of near-miss reports. A frequent reaction goes something like, "Wait ... we instituted this world-class error-reduction process and the result is ... we are getting more errors?!" Our response is, "No, those errors have been happening all along. The difference is that now people are speaking up about them, and we all have the chance to learn from them, so we don't have an accident!"

Clearly, the conversation following an incident-report or a near-miss conversation is of critical importance. We have both participated in developing a research-based body of knowledge about so-called after action reviews (AARs). In the military and among first responder groups, it is common practice for a team to get together after a mission/call and review their performance. Did they have the information they needed? Were they prepared with the proper equipment? As the situation they were addressing unfolded, were there emergent events that required them to adapt rapidly? If so, how did they respond? How did they communicate during the event? Most generally, what did they learn from their approach to the event that can help them be more effective in the future?

The logic of the AAR, and best practices in such post-event assessments, apply to incident/accident investigations and near-miss conversations in healthcare. Our experience with AARs in first responder groups tells us that conducting such reviews as a learning tool, and not as a blame game, improves performance, reduces errors going forward, and contributes to stronger teamwork and an overall more positive culture. Essentially, the AAR or debriefing can become a practical way for both teams and individuals to engage in ongoing reflection throughout their work and can help to mitigate errors and reduce accidents. When applied to the issue of burnout, we anticipate that those who use AARs or debriefings may discover new and innovative solutions to assist them in their efforts. We hope our readers will share their ideas with us as they engage in this worthy pursuit.

What Next? Living in the Next Normal (the COVID-19 Effect Revisited)

Throughout this book, there are sections at the conclusion of chapters describing how each of the various topics are impacted by COVID-19. Although this approach was initially motivated by the timing of writing the book, that is, in the early to middle part of the crisis, further reflection has led us to some additional conclusions.

First, at the time of writing this, the world was trying to get "back to normal," perhaps being a little hasty and overly ambitious in that effort, as cases continued to mount. And then came the surge of the Delta variant. Once the pandemic crisis subsides, the new normal, which we are calling the "next normal," is probably going to be one with a lot more hand sanitizer, masks, social distancing, and other precautions around illnesses in general. It is unlikely that the safety precautions we adopted out of necessity during the pandemic will ever completely go away, nor should they. We have all learned a lot about minimizing the spread of any virus. The next normal also comes with ongoing challenges for healthcare providers and physicians. It has always been a challenging, stressful profession, even in the best of times, but the next normal only makes that risk more visible to both the workers *and* the public. Living in this next normal will still require constant vigilance and reflection on how to best protect ourselves and each other, as well as provide the best care possible for patients.

Second, the coronavirus, like the many other viruses and illnesses that have plagued humanity for centuries, will indeed eventually subside, as we are seeing at the time of concluding our research and writing of this book. The demise of the coronavirus may come because pharmaceutical companies, physicians, and other healthcare providers develop effective vaccines and treatments and/or because for whatever reasons "herd immunity" gradually prevails. Then, the question will be, What happens next? When will the next big virus or worldwide health-related catastrophe hit? We can't know that. The question perhaps is, Will we be better prepared as individuals, teams, organizations, management, communities, and society? Will we be better able to manage our stress and reduce our risk of burnout? The answer, we hope, is "Yes." We can and must be more prepared. The strategies presented in this book can help us do just that.

Summing Up

In sum, the crisis of the burned-out physician is all too real. Many physicians are burned out, as are the other healthcare providers they work directly with. Their burnout obviously takes a toll on them, and it also puts their patient at risk. But we, all of us, can do something about it. In fact, we can do a lot about it if we better understand causes, symptoms, effects, and control strategies – solutions – as we have reviewed them here. We close this book with a heavy emphasis on self-reflection, taking AIM at key priorities, and incorporating the strategies of a learning organization.

Our hope and intention is that readers of this book who are in the healthcare enterprise develop a clearer understanding of the risks they face and find solutions they can implement and advocate for in order to reduce their risk of burnout, in general, but especially in the face of additional stresses brought on by the pandemic. Our hope and intention is that readers of this book who are patients develop a clearer understanding of the challenges their healthcare providers are under and become more proactive partners in co-managing their own healthcare.

Key Takeaways

- The workplace syndrome of burnout, resulting from excessive unmanaged stress on the job, is identified by exhaustion, depersonalization, and reduced effectiveness.
- Burnout is particularly prominent among physicians and other healthcare providers.
- One of the major consequences of physician burnout is increased likelihood of error.
- The burnout crisis in healthcare is a global issue, not limited to the United States.
- Solutions to address the burnout crisis range from broad governmental and professional society solutions to local organizational solutions to team and individual solutions.
- The highest-impact solutions are those at the level of national policy, which affect how organizations, teams, and individuals can operate.
- Prospective solutions at each level are reviewed, in a self-assessment format.
- The adaptive improvement model provides a simple, user-friendly format for identifying behaviors to continue, stop, or start in order to achieve improvements, in our case, reductions in burnout risk. It is presented with a worksheet for self-assessment.
- The contemporary concept of the "learning organization" is introduced and explained. Learning organizations scan the internal and external environment of their business, identify best-practice solutions that have been identified, and make sure those solutions are put into practice in their workplaces.
- Learning organizations capture and learn from incidents and from close calls, in part by using the after action review as a communication tool internally.

- The COVID-19 crisis has dramatically increased burnout risk among healthcare providers. When the pandemic is past and we are in the next normal, changes at all levels of the system must address the burnout crisis and reduce the risk for all healthcare providers and their patients.

REFERENCE

Wu, A. W., & Marks, C. M. (2013). Close calls in patient safety: Should we be paying closer attention? *CMAJ, 185*(13), 1119–1120.

Index

accident proneness, 76–77
Adaptive Improvement Model (AIM), 205–207
  AIM Worksheet, 205
  Continue, 205
  Start, 206
  Stop, 205–206
  Team Training Example, 207
advice, following and giving, 114–119
  comparisons of choices: physicians *vs.* patients, 114–115
  COVID-19 effect on, 118–119
  "do as I say, not as I do" by physicians: 114, 116
  need for physicians to follow advice given to patients, 118
  reluctance of medical providers in following: 96, 114
  safety knowledge *vs.* safe behavior disconnect, 116
  self-care/stress management advice, 95
advocacy/indirect actions for healthcare leaders, 173–174
Agency for Healthcare Research and Quality (AHRQ), 73–74
Agreeableness (Five Factor Model), 84
Alexander the Great, 123
American Medical Association (AMA)
  on benefits of continuing medical education, 152
  Chief Wellness Officer (CWO) roadmap, 176
  response to burnout crisis, 171–174
  workflow strategy recommendations, 161–162
American Psychological Association, 106–107
anger-hostility axis, 110
anxiety
  "cognitive reframing" therapy for, 90
  continuum of, 98
  from COVID-19 crisis: 25, 40, 78
  from flashbacks, 7
  in frontline healthcare workers, 40
  Neuroticism and, 84–85

Apple, 122
assistant physicians (APs), 61
attentional difficulties, 8
autonomic nervous system: 6, 14–15. *See also* fight or flight syndrome
aviation industry
  burnout in, 50
  CRM training programs: 49–50
  error management, 47–48

barriers
  to management practices for leaders, 174–176
  to a positive team culture, 155
  to proposed solutions in national healthcare, 196
  to proposed workflow solutions, 164
  to social support, 110–111
  to success, removal of, 152
bedside manner: 1, 13
behavioral symptoms, 5
best practices, for healthcare management, 169–171
  being adaptable, 171
  communication, 171
  COVID-19 pandemic effect, 171
  curiosity/openness to new tools, 170
  dedication to self-improvement, 171
  leading by example, 170–171
  reliance on the data, 170
  setting expectations, 170
big picture awareness, 140
bipolar disorder, 39
black box of decision-making, 116
British Medical Association, 38
Brown, P. A., 86
burnout, definitions
  common definitions: 1–2, 5, 199
  common symptoms, 199
  International Classification for Diseases, 2–3
  World Health Organization: 2, 6
burnout domino effect, 61

214

Printed by Printforce, United Kingdom